KW-050-724

SIBO COOKBOOK

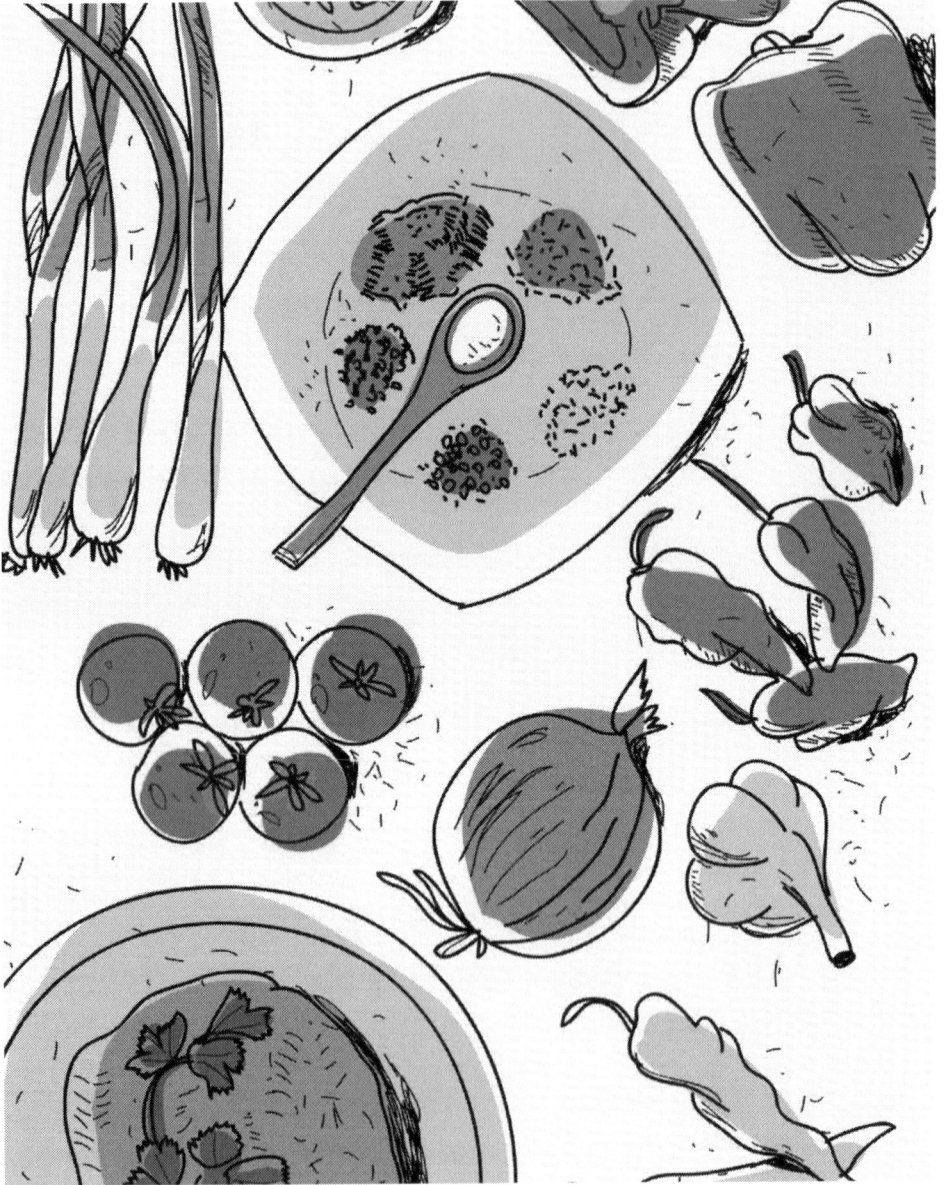

SIBO Cookbook

SIBO Diet Cookbook including 30 Day SIBO Diet Plan

Susan Mogan

LEGAL NOTICE

Copyright (c) 2019 by Susan Mogan

All rights are reserved. No portion of this book may be reproduced or duplicated using any form whether mechanical, electronic, or otherwise. No portion of this book may be transmitted, stored in a retrieval database, or otherwise made available in any manner whether public or private unless specific permission is granted by the publisher. Vector illustration credit: vecteezy.com

This book does not offer advice, but merely provides information. The author offers no advice whether medical, financial, legal, or otherwise, nor does the author encourage any person to pursue any specific course of action discussed in this book. This book is not a substitute for professional advice. The reader accepts complete and sole responsibility for the manner in which this book and its contents are used. The publisher and the author will not be held liable for any damages caused.

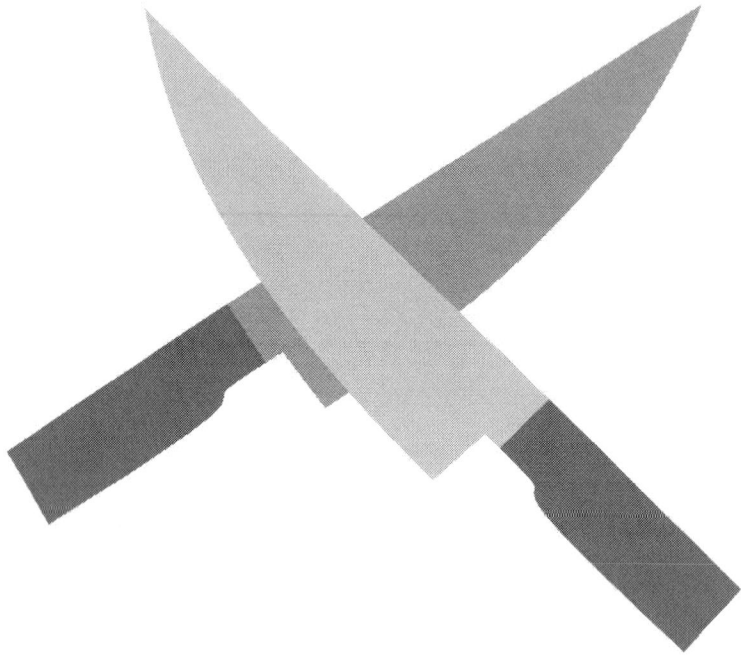

CONTENTS

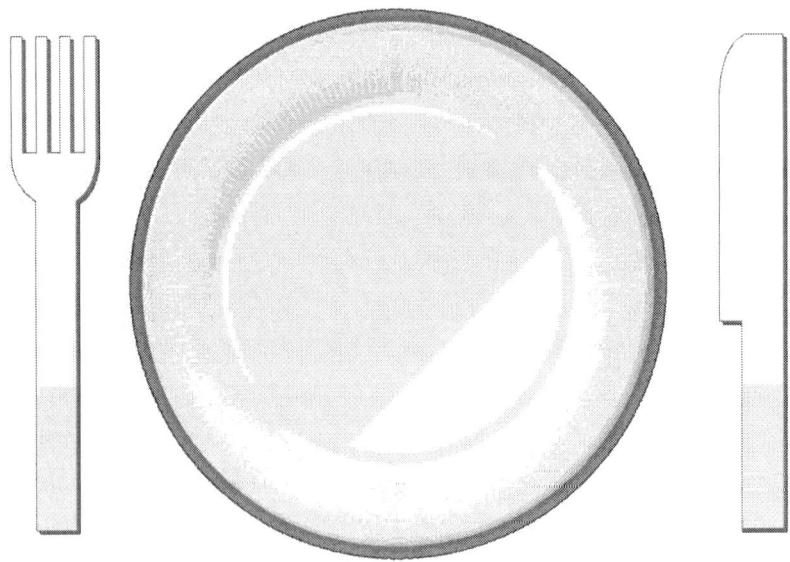

FORWARD: HOW CHANGING MY DIET CHANGED MY LIFE

For years, I struggled with stomach and digestion issues, and couldn't figure out why. I couldn't enjoy common foods and no matter what I ate, I started out every day feeling okay, but by the end of it, I felt like a hot air balloon because the bloating was so bad. Going out to eat was a nightmare because I never knew what would trigger the worst of my symptoms, so food caused me a lot of anxiety. Finally, I read about SIBO (small intestinal bacterial overgrowth) and instantly felt vindicated. It wasn't just in my head! There's supposed to be bacteria in the human gut, but there was too much in mine, and it was causing inflammation and stealing nutrition from the food I ate. What I was experiencing wasn't "normal" for me; there was actually something wrong.

After talking to my doctor about what could be causing my SIBO, I started out on a course of antibiotics. This was to destroy the high levels of harmful bacteria in my system, but I wasn't on them very long. Antibiotics can actually cause SIBO because they don't distinguish between good and bad bacteria; they just destroy everything. I learned it's important to replenish the good bacteria with foods like Greek yogurt, but a probiotic supplement might not be the best answer. I chose to eat probiotic foods.

Antibiotics were just the beginning of my treatment. The real challenge was to design a diet that could give me the nutrition I needed while letting my body heal. There are a variety of diets, but all of them restrict carbs and dairy. I also cut out *all* sugar and processed foods. A high fat, high salt, and high sugar diet wreaks havoc on the digestive system, so I needed to be very strict. I thought cooking would be difficult, but I actually found a lot of recipes and resources that made it relatively easy. The whole point of SIBO diets is to keep meals simple with a few key ingredients, so I never spend too much time in the kitchen.

My life has changed so much since I discovered I had SIBO. I've been able to identify the foods that cause the most symptoms (dairy and certain vegetables), so now I can avoid them. Keeping these out of my system lets me eat a wider variety of foods symptom-free, whereas before, it felt like I couldn't eat anything without getting sick. I still don't eat processed foods or foods high in sugar, and my health has improved so much. I have more energy, I'm at a healthy weight, and my anxiety is gone. That doesn't mean I can't treat myself; because my gut is balanced, small amounts of sugar don't aggravate me like before. If you've been experiencing symptoms like I was, you don't have to endure that life anymore. You can find healing and freedom, and transform your relationship with food!

Sincerely,
Karen Diaz

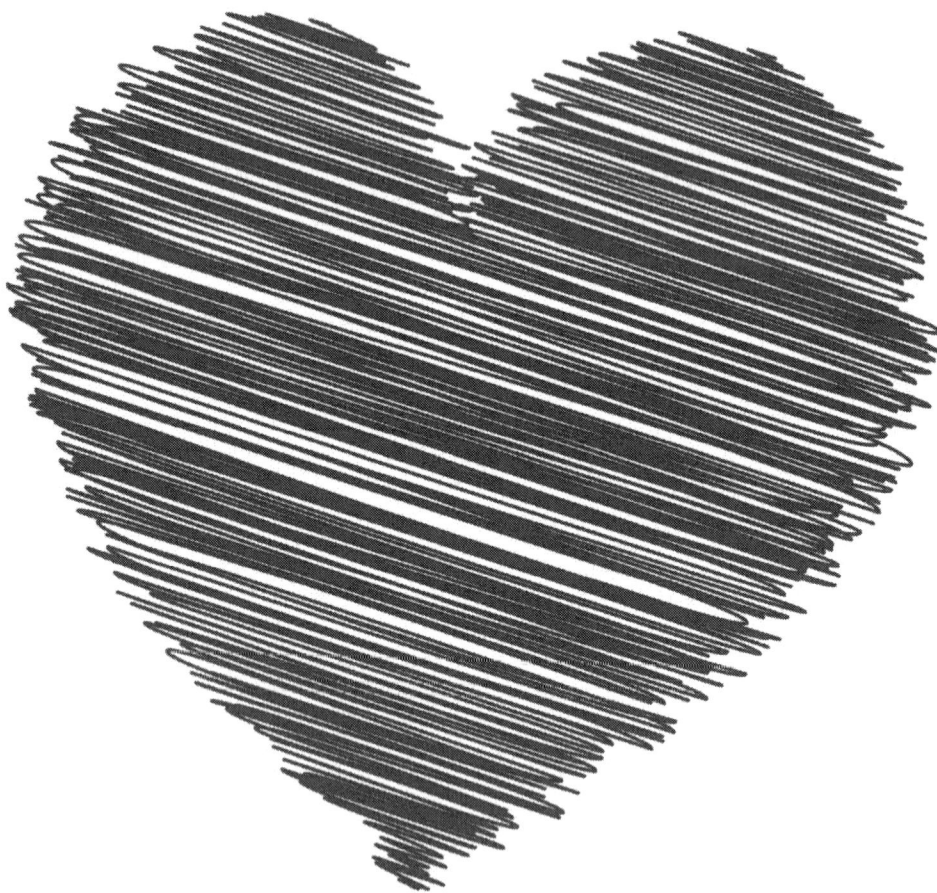

A NOTE FROM THE AUTHOR

There's been a lot of research lately into the human "gut," or digestive system. Scientists have learned that it is home to a wide variety of bacteria, some harmful, and some beneficial. This is significant because the digestive system makes up 80% of the body's immune system, so if there's something wrong with your gut, your overall health is affected. When that balance of bacteria gets out of whack, it can cause what's known as SIBO, or small intestinal bacterial overgrowth. Harmful bacteria begins eating the nutrition your body needs, leaving you with less. This leads to digestive tract inflammation and malnutrition. If untreated, all of your organs and bodily functions begin to fail.

How do you know if you have SIBO? There are lots of warnings signs and unpleasant symptoms. Constipation, diarrhea, chronic bloating, food sensitivities, nausea, and vomiting are common. You might also suffer from allergies, skin problems, anxiety, and depression. Eating becomes a minefield and you never know what might aggravate your sensitive gut. Thankfully, there are steps you can take to reduce your symptoms and heal from what is essentially an infection.

In this book, you'll learn more about what causes SIBO and how to treat it. A change in diet is the most important change you can make. There are four major eating lifestyles that doctors might recommend. They vary in restrictiveness and what specific foods to avoid, but in general, they all involve restricting or cutting out carbs and dairy. You might also cut out grains. All diets have you cut out sugar and processed food, which is the ideal fuel for harmful bacteria. Giving your digestive tract and system a break from aggravating foods lets it heal, and then you can begin enjoying a wider variety of food without symptoms.

There are other tips that can make SIBO recovery easier, such as taking vitamins, antibiotics, and eating probiotic foods. You should wait longer between meals to give the body time to digest properly and avoid snacking, since your digestive system needs a break. Eating out will be trickier when you're starting on your diet, so it's best to cook at home. Equipment like a rice cooker, slow cooker, and immersion blender makes cooking convenient. Once you are able to eat at restaurants, always look at menus beforehand and have a list of SIBO-friendly places you can recommend to friends.

The ultimate goal of any SIBO diet is three-fold: decrease the amount of bacteria in your system, let your body heal, and eat diverse, nutrition-rich foods. Anything processed or artificial is like poison to your body, so stay away. Whole, real foods are not only healthy for you, they taste better. This recipe book proves that you can still eat well while treating SIBO and ultimately recovering from it. You don't have to live in constant fear and anxiety about triggering a bout of symptoms without understanding why. Learn what causes your symptoms and then cut them out of your diet. With those gone, other food won't aggravate your healed system. You can find freedom and enjoyment in food, maybe for the first time in your life.

You deserve it!
Susan Mogan

INTRODUCTION

If you haven't heard of SIBO, you're not alone. SIBO, which stands for small intestinal bacterial overgrowth, is not a well-used term in the medical community, but it may be way more common than previously-thought. It's underdiagnosed because it bears a lot of similarities with conditions like IBS and Crohn's. It's also closely-related to what's known as Candida, a yeast fungus that usually helps with digestion and nutrient absorption. When there's too much of it in the system, it breaks down the intestinal lining, gets into the bloodstream, and releases toxins. Leaky gut syndrome often follows. The main difference between Candida and SIBO is that SIBO involves a variety of bacteria, not just yeast.

SIBO should be taken seriously because it can lead to malnutrition, which in turn leads to widespread organ and function failure. Without sufficient nutrients, the body begins to break down and fail. In this introduction, we will go over symptoms of SIBO, its causes, and diets that doctors recommend to treat it. You'll see what foods you are allowed to eat and which ones aggravate SIBO. We'll also discuss the significance of supplements like vitamins and antibiotics. Before getting to the recipe portion of this book, you'll learn what kitchen supplies you need and some helpful tips that other SIBO patients and experts have shared. Recovery is within reach; you don't have to live your life afraid of food.

I. WHAT IS SIBO?

If you've struggled with digestive issues like nausea, chronic bloating, and constipation on top of food sensitivities, headaches, fatigue, and joint pain, you might have SIBO. Full name "small intestinal bacterial overgrowth," SIBO refers to a bacterial excess in your small intestine. Ordinarily, your small bowel gets rid of everything - leftover food, digestive enzymes, and excessive bacteria - every two hours. However, if this sweep doesn't happen, your small intestine (SI) can't get rid of the bacteria and you've got SIBO. For years, SIBO wasn't even recognized as a real condition, but a high number of people have it, especially those with IBS.

Symptoms

SIBO comes with a nasty checklist of symptoms affecting your gut and the rest of your body. Chronic bloating, gas, belching, stomach cramping, diarrhea, and constipation are common. So is nausea, heartburn, and acid reflux. You will be more sensitive to foods and experience fatigue. SIBO can also cause seemingly-unrelated issues like headaches, joint pain, asthma, skin problems, and depression and anxiety.

SIBO's most serious consequence is malnutrition. The excessive bacteria in your SI eats all the nutrition that your body needs, so every organ is affected. You can become deficient in vitamin B12, which is essential for your neurological system. Other lost nutrients include iron, niacin, thiamine, vitamin K, and vitamin A.

SIBO occurs when your small intestine has too much bacteria, preventing adequate nutrition absorption and triggering unpleasant symptoms. These include diarrhea, constipation, chronic bloating and gas, food sensitivities, fatigue, and more.

Getting tested

Doctors test for SIBO with a breath test. You don't need to give any blood or stool samples. The breath test measures methane or hydrogen in your breath, since these are a result of bacteria breaking down sugar in the body. If the test shows you have SIBO, doctors will consider what might be causing it.

Potential SIBO causes

There are several possible explanations for SIBO:

Slow SI movement

SIBO can be caused by what's known officially as "small intestine dysmotility." This means your SI is performing at a slower rate than it should. Genetics, autoimmune problems, or an inflamed GI tract could be to blame.

Slow bowels

When it takes your body more than 72 days to produce a bowel movement following eating, bacteria gets a chance to build up in your SI.

Pre-existing medical conditions

Certain conditions like Type 2 diabetes, leaky gut syndrome, and celiac disease increase a person's risk for SIBO. Crohn's can also cause SIBO if you have an untreated bowel obstruction for too long. Any medical issue involving the gut's muscle function can lead to SIBO.

Certain medications

The excessive use of medications like antidepressants, birth control, antacids, and antibiotics might play a role in damaging the SI and bowels. They interfere with the body's balance of harmful and beneficial bacteria.

Your diet

It makes sense that diet and SIBO are closely-related. Studies have suggested that alcohol might play a big role, even if you only drink moderately. Refined sugar also feeds bacteria so it grow in excess. Too much yeast (found in gluten) causes leaky gut syndrome, which is usually paired with SIBO. If you have leaky gut or SIBO, you are at a significant risk for getting the other as well.

Not enough stomach acid

Your stomach acid regulates the amount of bacteria in your gut, but if you have too little acid, that bacteria grows unchecked. Factors like lots of processed food or age contribute to low stomach acid. Doctors find that most SIBO cases are associated with low stomach acid.

> **SIBO can be caused by other gut conditions like IBS, Type 2 diabetes, and Crohn's Disease. It can also be triggered by an insufficient amount of stomach acid, a poor diet, certain medications, or slow bowels and slow SI movement.**

II. DIETS

SIBO treatment will always include a change in diet. Your SI and digestive tract are being traumatized by the food you eat, and without time to heal, the problems just get worse. There are a handful of diets that doctors might recommend designed to cut out hard-to-digest foods and foods that aggravate the system, while adding in foods known for their healing properties. Here are four you will hear about most:

Specific Carbohydrate Diet (SCD)

Developed by a doctor and biochemist, the SCD has been tested for more than half a century. It has a very high success rate for those with Crohn's, celiac, chronic diarrhea, and similar diseases. Because SIBO also affects the gut, SCD is often recommended for the condition. The diet works by eliminating complex carbs (disaccharides and polysaccharides) because these carbs are not easily digested *and* they feed bacteria. By cutting out their fuel, the bacteria dies. SCD also restricts fiber when you first start out, so your intestinal wall can heal. It's considered the most restrictive diet for SIBO and requires the most work.

Here's what you are *allowed* to eat:

- Unprocessed meats (chicken, pork, beef, fish)
- Eggs
- Certain dairy (natural cheddar, Colby, swiss, gruyere, homemade 24-hour yogurt)
- Non-starchy vegetables (cucumber, celery, asparagus, beets, carrots, mushrooms, leeks spinach, lettuce, squash, etc)
- Fresh fruit
- Nuts
- Fresh-squeezed fruit juice w/ no added sugar
- Almond milk
- Nut flour
- Certain alcohol (gin, scotch, dry wines, whisky, vodka)
- Honey
- Spices and condiments w/out starch or sugar

Since SCD is a restrictive diet, there are a lot of foods you cannot eat:

- All processed meats
- Certain dairy (milk, ice cream, mozzarella, ricotta, feta)
- Starchy vegetables (potatoes, yams, okra, parsnips, chickpeas, bean sprouts, seaweed)
- Plantains
- Dried fruit with added starch and sugar
- All grains and flours
- Soy milk
- Certain alcohol (beer, brandy, sake, sherry, port)
- Spices/condiments w/ added sugar or starch
- Maple syrup
- Chocolate

Low FODMAP Diet (LFD)

FODMAP stands for "fermentable oligo-di-monosaccharides and polyols." These compounds exist in certain foods in high or low amounts. The higher the FODMAP content, the worse they are for those with IBS and SIBO. Foods high in FODMAP are harder to digest and absorb, which gives bacteria time to ferment them and cause SIBO symptoms. When you begin the Low FODMAP diet, you must cut down on foods highest in FODMAP and then slowly reintroduce them if it seems like a good idea. This process can last anywhere from two weeks to two months. LFD is considered moderately-restrictive.

What this diet does is remove the highest sources of sugar. The sugar in foods like dairy, grains, and many vegetables and fruit are harder for the body to absorb. They irritate your gut. Restricting them gives the body time to heal, so you may be able to add some of the higher FODMAP foods back into your diet. Studies support Low FODMAP for both SIBO and IBS, making it one of the most common recommended diets for the condition.

The three phases

There are three phases in this diet: elimination, reintroduction, and maintenance. The elimination phase cuts out as many high FODMAP foods as possible so you can see if your SIBO improves at all. This will let you know if FODMAP foods are responsible for your issues. The next phase - reintroduction - has you gradually add higher FODMAP foods back in and see how your body responds. If your symptoms flare up again, you'll know what specific foods you need to keep out of your diet. The maintenance phase is just the term for your new and improved long-term diet. You'll know what foods you should avoid and which are okay.

So, what should you eat and what should you avoid on the LFD diet?

Here's a list of low FODMAP foods, which are acceptable during all three phases:

- Meat (Chicken, fish, pork, turkey, beef)
- Eggs
- Lactose-free dairy

- Nut milks
- Wheat-free grains
- Vegetables (cucumbers, carrots, dark leafy greens, squash, corn, mushrooms, potatoes, etc)
- One serving of fruit per day (berries, bananas, tropical fruits, citrus fruits)
- Herbs (mint, sage, thyme, cilantro)
- Seasonings (salt, pepper)
- Condiments (mayo, broth, mustard)
- Maple syrup
- Balsamic vinegar
- Olive oil
- Vanilla extract
- Dark chocolate

As for foods you should avoid on the LFD diet, there are also quite a few:

- Dairy (cottage cheese, ice cream, yogurt, sour cream, anything with lactose)
- Coconut (coconut cream, coconut milk)
- Soy products
- Beans
- Grains (wheat, flour, barley, rye, etc)
- Certain vegetables (artichokes, broccoli, sun-dried tomatoes, brussel sprouts, onion, garlic, asparagus, beets, cabbage, fennel, okra, snow peas)
- Fruit in excess (especially apples, apricots, avocado, dates, cherries, dried fruit, canned fruit, prunes, plums, nectarines, peaches, watermelon)
- Seasonings/spices (garlic powder, onion powder, jams, jellies)
- Artificial seasonings
- Honey and sugar
- Pickles and pickle relish
- Fruit and vegetable juice

There are four diets that doctors might recommend for treating SIBO: The Specific Carb Diet, Low FODMAP Diet, Cedars Sinai-Low Fermentation Diet, and the GAPS Diet. They vary in restrictiveness, but in general, you eliminate or cut down significantly on grains, dairy, fruit, and certain vegetables. You'll also eliminate all processed and artificial foods.

Cedars Sinai-Low Fermentation Diet

Developed at Cedars Sinai in LA, this diet is all about spacing out your meals and eating low-fermentation foods. You are allowed to eat easily-digested sugars and starches, so it's less restrictive than other SIBO diets. You cannot have any lactose, however, or foods high in fiber. The tricky aspect of the Cedars Sinai diet is that you aren't allowed to snack. No grazing gives your body time to digest and absorb foods properly.

You are allowed to eat:

- All proteins
- Lactose-free dairy
- Rice
- Potatoes
- French, sourdough, and white bread
- Root vegetables (carrots, potatoes, yams, cucumbers, squash, zucchini)
- Tomatoes
- Bell peppers
- Small amounts of fruit
- Water, tea, and coffee

You cannot eat:

- Any foods with lactose, including milk
- Whole-wheat or high-fiber bread
- Certain vegetables (beans, cabbage, broccoli, cauliflower, leafy vegetables, legumes)
- A lot of fruit
- Anything with Splenda or sucralose

Gut and Psychology Syndrome Diet (GAPS)

This phase-filled diet is derived from the Specific Carbs Diet. The general goal is to remove hard-to-digest foods and replace them with nutrient-dense ones that allow the intestinal lining to heal. It has a three-part "protocol," or outline for success no matter where you are in the diet. The Nutritional protocol requires the elimination of all refined and processed carbs; the Supplementation protocol usually means taking a probiotic; while finally, the Detoxification protocol means cleaning the liver and colon of toxins.

The parts

GAPS itself is broken into two parts: the Introduction diet and Full GAPS. The Introduction diet is very restrictive and challenging. If you have severe SIBO, starting out with the Introduction is usually recommended, but if your symptoms aren't too bad, going right into the Full GAPs and focusing on the protocols might be more beneficial.

The Introduction has six stages that can take patients 3-6 weeks to complete, though it really depends on the specific person. The Introduction's goal is to reduce SIBO symptoms quickly and jumpstart gut healing. Foods include homemade stock, ginger tea, probiotic foods, and so on. Different foods are added throughout each stage.

Once all six stages are done, you move to the Full GAPS diet. Most of your eating consists of organic meat, fish, eggs, vegetables, and fermented foods. For best results, follow the Full Gaps for 18-24 months. Natural fats and a cup of bone broth should be included with every meal, since they help lubricate and heal the gut.

Here's a sample list of foods you'll be eating:

- Meat (beef, chicken, fish, pork)
- Eggs
- Certain vegetables (asparagus, artichoke, spinach, squash, etc)
- Certain fruit (apples, berries, ripe bananas, apricots, melons, mangos)
- Olive oil
- Coconut oil
- Butter and ghee
- Fresh coconut milk
- Natural honey
- Homemade yogurt
- Nuts (pecans, almonds, cashews, etc)
- Cheese
- High-quality spices
- Nut flours

The list for foods you can't eat is also quite long, so we'll abbreviate it:

- Baked beans
- Cottage cheese
- Buttermilk
- Cream
- Butter substitutes
- Barley
- Grain flour
- Balsamic vinegar
- White potatoes
- Sweet potatoes
- Pasta
- Rice
- Cornstarch
- Oats
- Sugar (includes agave and molasses)
- Chocolate
- Soda pop
- All processed meats (ham, bologna, salted and preserved fish)

Which diet should you try?

There are other diets designed for SIBO, but most are variations or combinations of the main four we discussed. How do you know which one works for you? Most people are going to recover well on a low FODMAP diet. It's relatively simple and not overly-restrictive. If your SIBO is more severe, you might need to cut out grains and starch, and go on a SCD diet.

No matter who you are, it's a good idea to try the FODMAP diet first and then modify it based on your condition. Work with your doctor to figure out what works and what doesn't.

The diet you choose should meet three goals: Decrease the bacteria in your system while increasing your body's ability to absorb nutrients; give your body time to heal itself; and achieve a balanced, healthy diet with food diversity.

Lifestyle changes

What are you doing differently when you change your diet to curb SIBO? There are a handful of tips to remember that can make the process easier and ensure your body heals the way it's supposed to, no matter which specific diet you choose:

Wait longer between meals

Many doctors recommend what's known as intermittent fasting. You don't go a day without food, but you do eat only two meals a day with at least 14 hours between your dinner and breakfast the next morning. Some people eat three meals a day with 4-5 hours between breakfast to lunch and lunch to dinner. It depends on what works for you. This fasting lets your body go through the digestion process thoroughly. Timing out your meals this way is especially good if your SIBO causes chronic constipation.

Eat slowly and chew thoroughly

When we say chew slowly and thoroughly, we mean *really* slowly and thoroughly. As in, it will feel weird and take practice to do right. You want to chew your food until it has become mush. This will make it easier for your body to digest and absorb the nutrients you need. Eating soft, well-cooked foods as well as meals like soup makes this chewing challenge easier.

Stop snacking

Constant eating is arguably the worst thing you can do when you're trying to get over SIBO. Your digestive system never gets a rest or a chance to heal. Even if it's a small piece of food, it can sabotage your recovery. You want to be really consistent about eating nutritious meals on a schedule. If you're getting hungry just two hours after a meal, you need to consider what you ate. Maybe it didn't include enough protein and fiber. If you're eating healthy meals with protein, healthy fats, fiber, and all the nutrients you need, you shouldn't feel the cravings and hunger pangs that cause snacking.

Stop eating processed foods

The biggest lifestyle change for most people with SIBO is stopping the processed foods completely. There's really nothing good we can say about processed food, junk food, and fast food. These foods are high in all the bad things - unhealthy fat, salt, and sugar. They are also very low in nutrients and enzymes needed for digestion. High fat and salt are very damaging to your digestive tract, triggering symptoms like constipation. The consequences go beyond your gut and digestion, too. An Oregon

State University study showed that a high-fat and high-sugar diet can be so destructive to your gut bacteria, it actually lowers your cognitive abilities.

Stop taking antacids and proton pump inhibitors

Lowering the amount of stomach acid in your system by taking antacids and proton pump inhibitors makes digestion harder. You want stomach acid to kill harmful bacteria and protect your small intestine. You probably know what antacids are, but proton pump inhibitors include drugs like Prilosec, Dexilant, Prevacid, Nexium, Vimovo, and Zegerid.

> **To reduce your SIBO symptoms, change your lifestyle so you wait longer between meals, chew thoroughly, stop snacking or eating processed foods, eliminate antacids and medications like Prilosec, and drink more water.**

Drink more water

Drinking enough water is critical to your SIBO recovery. It keeps your digestive system running smoothly, and if your SIBO symptoms include diarrhea, you need to be replenishing your liquids to avoid dehydration. Some doctors will recommend not drinking a lot of water before, during, and directly after a meal, because you need all your stomach acid for digestion. Since plain water can be boring and you might need more nutrients to fight malnutrition, water with slices of citrus (lemon and lime), cucumber, and weak herbal teas can help you get more vitamins into your body. Good teas include rosehip, rooibos, peppermint, ginger, hibiscus, white tea, green tea, and weak dandelion tea. You should *not* drink chamomile, oolong, or licorice.

III. VITAMIN SUPPLEMENTS, ANTIBIOTICS, AND PROBIOTICS

It takes more than a change in diet to treat SIBO, especially if it's serious. Supplements, antibiotics, and probiotics will come up in your research and are often recommended by doctors, so it's important to discuss their merits.

Vitamin supplements

Taking vitamin supplements makes sense when you have SIBO, because your body isn't absorbing the nutrients it needs from food. You will most likely have to take vitamin B12, vitamin K, vitamin D, iron, and zinc.

B12 - Your body needs B12 to make red blood cells, which take oxygen to your body. Without enough B12, you'll be weak and fatigued.

K - It transports calcium through your blood and helps blood clot properly.

D - Vitamin D helps your body absorb calcium, so your bones can grow and stay strong.

Iron - Iron is necessary for proper blood production. 70% of your body's iron is found in red blood cells.

<u>Zinc</u> - Your immune system needs zinc to work, while your cells need it to divide and grow. It's also necessary for your senses of smell and taste.

Antibiotics

Because SIBO is caused by an overgrowth of bacteria, many think that they need antibiotics to destroy this bacteria. It's often the first thing that's prescribed along with diet. Rifaximin is the most studied and studies show a 50% improvement in just one week, while a combination of rifaximin and neomycin is 85% successful after 10 days.

Antibiotics should not be used for the long-term, however. They're good at destroying excess bacteria right away, but they can't distinguish between good and harmful bacteria, and they don't address SIBO's cause. When scientists looked at SIBO and antibiotics in the long-term, most patients need to be retreated because SIBO keeps coming back. This is bad news because going on antibiotics again and again can make your body resistant. Intestinal bacteria is especially good at adapting, so many doctors now avoid antibiotics completely if they can and instead focus on diet.

Many SIBO patients also use herbal or natural antibiotics, which are plant-derived extracts known for their antibacterial qualities. Think garlic, which is arguably the world's first antibiotic. These are not as strong as their synthetic cousins, however, so herbs need to be used in blends with one another to keep up. There's also not very much research about their effectiveness.

Probiotics

Probiotics are defined as live bacteria and yeasts, so why would you take this to cure SIBO? Isn't that counterintuitive? Probiotics are *good* bacteria and help with healing the body while other measures help decrease the amount of harmful bacteria. However, probiotics are a hot topic in SIBO treatment and may not be helpful for everyone. Sometimes they even make symptoms worse. One study shows that a probiotic with Lactobacillus casei did *not* help reduce SIBO symptoms, but research continues. Doctors may recommend probiotic foods like yogurt and kefir after antibiotics because your gut is low in good bacteria, but these should always be introduced slowly.

> **Vitamins and antibiotics will most likely be part of your SIBO recovery, though you should never take antibiotics long-term. Probiotics are more controversial and may make your symptoms worse. Consult your doctor before eating probiotic food or taking a supplement.**

IV. KITCHEN SUPPLIES

When you're treating SIBO, you'll be doing most if not all of your cooking at home. Going out to eat is fraught with unknowns about ingredients, and portion sizes are usually too large for your healing gut. There are tips on how to eat at restaurants with SIBO, and we'll go over those in the next section. However, this is a cookbook, so let's explore what kitchen supplies you'll need to make SIBO-friendly recipes:

Tea kettle

In addition to water, you will probably be drinking a variety of teas. Having a good tea kettle lets you heat up water to the right temperatures very quickly. Bear in mind that different teas have different recommended temperatures. For example, some herbal teas shouldn't be steeped in boiling water, while others are. Green tea is typically made at a lower temperature or it becomes too "grassy" and bitter.

Tea infuser

Speaking of tea, getting a tea infuser is also a good idea. You'll be making teas from leaves, since bagged teas are typically not the best quality. Infusers let you steep leaves in water, and then easily remove the leaf waste without needing to pour your tea through a strainer. There are three main types of infusers: baskets, balls, and silicone balls. Baskets have the most space, which many say they produce the best tea flavor. Balls are more compact, so you don't have any teeny residual leaves in your brew, but the flavor isn't as full. The same thing happens with silicone infusers, and some drinkers say there's a weird taste leftover. If you really care about getting the best tea flavor, go with a basket.

Immersion blender

Immersion blenders (also called "stick" blenders) are extremely convenient. You can puree meals like soups in their cooking pots, so you don't need to bother with a heavy blender that needs to be cleaned separately. They're also way cheaper than regular blenders with some costing under $20. If you plan on using your immersion blender a lot, you'll probably want to spend more around $30-$40 to get the power and durability you need. Some blenders also come with blending jars for smoothies. Most are pretty small, however, and fit just two ingredients for a smoothie that serves one.

Good measuring spoons and cups

You probably have a set or two of measuring spoons and cups, but if you don't, you should get some before starting out on your SIBO diet. When you have SIBO, you cook mostly at home, so good measurement equipment is essential. Find ones that are easy to clean and durable, so they don't start peeling or chipping with frequent runs in the dishwasher. Stainless steel is always a good choice for both spoons and cups. You should also get a separate measuring cup for liquids that has easy-to-read gradations, so the measurements are always accurate. You can typically choose between glass or plastic with liquid measuring cups.

Rice cooker

Some of the SIBO-recommended diets let you eat rice, so a dedicated rice cooker is a great purchase. You pick the best size for your needs, so you can make batches that last a few days.

> **Kitchen supplies like a good tea kettle and infuser, rice cooker, and nutritional app can make cooking with SIBO much easier.**

Slow cooker or pressure cooker

In addition to a rice cooker (or instead of, if the appliance has a "Rice" function), a slow cooker or pressure cooker is a great investment. You can cook meals overnight or during the day with very little hands-on work, and the foods will be cooked thoroughly for your SIBO needs. Pressure cookers are having a big moment, especially the Instant Pot brand, and you can cook virtually anything in them. They also have a slow cooker function, so you're getting multiple functions in one device.

Nutritional app

When you have SIBO, it's important to keep track of what you're eating, so you can figure out if you need more of a certain food to get the nutrition you need. Nutritional apps like MyFitnessPal are a great way to track your eating habits, and you don't have to spend a lot of time adding together your calories and nutritional macros. You can even find apps devoted to specific diets.

V. How to go out to eat with SIBO

Going out to a restaurant with friends or family should be a fun experience, but when you have SIBO, it can be really frustrating and generate anxiety. What if you eat the wrong thing and end up sick? Or are you just never going to be able to out ever again? You *can* still go out; you just have to employ smart strategies and make good choices. Here are some helpful tips on how to eat the right food and avoid dishes that trigger symptoms:

Look at menus beforehand

The #1 must-do when it comes to eating out with SIBO is to look at menus *beforehand*. It's very stressful to be at dinner and look at the menu for the first time, and realize you have no idea what you can eat. When you're planning, have a few specific places in mind and look at their menus online. Pick some options you can eat and see if the restaurant allows for substitutions.

Have places you know are SIBO-friendly

When someone asks you out to eat, have some places in mind. This way, if they suggest a place you know you can't go to, you can say, "What about this place instead?" It's more convenient and considerate than having your friend try to list off places. Once you have specific places you know are acceptable, you can rely on them in the future and don't always have to start researching whenever you want to go out.

Stay simple

The best strategy for eating at restaurants when you have SIBO is to keep things simple. A meal should consist of a protein and side. You know you can eat lean meats like chicken, fish, beef, pork, and so on. Sides like mushrooms, dark leafy greens, and potatoes are acceptable, depending on the diet you're following. If a dish has a sauce you aren't sure about, just ask for the meal without it. The more basic a dish, the easier it is to know what the ingredients are.

When eating out with SIBO, always look at menus beforehand and keep a list of SIBO-friendly places to suggest to friends. When you're choosing a meal, keep things as simple as possible and remember to relax.

You don't need to be perfect

A little sugar or other higher FODMAP foods in small amounts probably won't trigger your worst symptoms. When you're first starting on recovery, you want to be pretty strict, but when it's been a while and you're ready to start eating out again, it's okay to not always stick to your diet 100%. There will be certain foods you can't have, no matter what amount, but there are others that are only a problem if you eat too much. Eating out at a restaurant should be a fun, relaxing experience, so make good choices, but don't worry too much about every single ingredient.

VI. TIPS FROM EXPERTS AND THOSE WITH SIBO

SIBO is more common than previously thought, and the internet is home to all sorts of blogs and articles written on the subject. We collected some of the best advice we found from those with SIBO and doctors who see SIBO patients:

Drink lemon water before eating

Before eating a meal, drinking 8-ounces of water with 2 tablespoons of fresh lemon juice can help stimulate your stomach acid, which will make digestion easier. Lemons have lots of vitamins great for gut health, including vitamin C and fiber. Pectin, a fiber, helps promote healthy gut bacteria, so if you're concerned about a treatment of antibiotics doing *too* good job a job, adding lemon water to your diet can help encourage good bacteria growth.

Always have a bottle of water with you

We talked about how important hydration is for SIBO recovery, so one of the most common tips is to always carry a water bottle with you. Find a durable, BPA-free one that is convenient and portable for wherever you go. Some even have diffusers in them for fruit and herbs. If you have trouble keeping track of how much water you drink, get a water bottle with gradations on it.

Try collagen supplements

On the GAPS diet, you'll be drinking a lot of bone broth. Why? Bone broth is packed with valuable amino acids and collagen, which studies show can help repair and grow cells. Your inflamed intestinal lining could use that cell-regenerating power. Even if you aren't on the GAPS diet, consider adding bone broth or a collagen supplement. You can buy collagen peptides or collagen protein powder to mix into smoothies, soups, sauces, and more. When you drink bone broth, you want to make your own from scratch because commercial brands often include spices like garlic and preservatives. Talk to your doctor to see if collagen is something that could help you.

Eat small portions

A certain food may be fine for you in small amounts, but as soon as you overeat, your SIBO symptoms start. To be safe, eat a variety of foods in small portions when you're starting out so you can figure out what you're most sensitive to. As your symptoms subside and your body heals, you'll have a much better grasp on what amounts are acceptable for you.

Avoid anything that's not "real"

A good rule of thumb for any SIBO diet is avoiding anything that isn't real. This is especially important when it comes to artificial sweeteners. These can aggravate SIBO symptoms in extreme ways and potentially disrupt other bodily functions. When you're shopping at the store for food, always read ingredient labels and familiarize yourself with artificial stuff like BHA, BHT, sodium nitrate, artificial colors, propyl gallate, and aspartame.

> **Those with SIBO and experts on the condition recommend tips like always carrying a water bottle with you, eating small portions, drinking lemon water to stimulate stomach acid, and being careful about how much fruit you eat.**

Be cautious of fruit

Fruit is a real, whole food, but that doesn't mean it's all healthy. Fruit is naturally high in fructose, which can be big symptom-trigger for those with SIBO. Excess fructose stays in your gut and the body frequently can't digest it properly. This is known as fructose malabsorption. All that fructose is prime feeding for gut bacteria *and* since fructose attracts water, it can trigger really bad diarrhea. Avoid fruits high in fructose and stick to low-glycemic berries, grapefruit, and Granny Smith apples. When your symptoms get better and you've healed, it's okay to eat a banana or other higher-glycemic fruit once and a while if you can tolerate it, but you really want to use caution.

VII. SUMMARIZING EVERYTHING

In this introduction, we covered all the basics of what SIBO is and how it manifests in people. SIBO stands for "small intestinal bacterial overgrowth," and occurs for a number of reasons, including insufficient stomach acid, certain medications, and existing conditions like IBS or Crohn's. What happens is that harmful gut bacteria outnumbers the good bacteria, causing an imbalance in your gut that affects your immune system and eventually, your whole body. Symptoms include gastric distress (constipation and/or diarrhea), painful gas and chronic bloating, nausea and vomiting following meals, fatigue, and other problems like depression and anxiety. Not treating SIBO can lead to malnutrition.

Diets

One of the best treatments for SIBO is a change in diet. This puts your symptoms on hold and lets your body heal. We covered four diets: the Specific Carb Diet, Low FODMAP Diet, Cedars Sinai-Low Fermentation, and the Gut and Psychology Syndrome Diet (known more commonly as GAPS). Here's a brief outline of what each diet requires:

The Specific Carb Diet

- A very restrictive diet, can be challenging
- Eliminates complex carbs
- Restricts fiber
- No grains allowed

Low FODMAP

- Moderately-restrictive
- Eliminates grains and dairy
- Consists of three phases
- Intended for the long-term

Cedars Sinai

- The least restrictive diet
- Eliminates dairy
- All about spacing out your food

GAPS

- Based on the Specific Carb Diet
- Has the most phases
- Eliminates some grain and dairy

No matter what diet you choose, the goals are to give your body the time and opportunity to heal, to figure out what foods you can tolerate and which foods you can't, and to make your diet as diverse as possible.

Additional treatments

We also covered additional treatments briefly in the introduction, specifically vitamins, antibiotics, and probiotics. Vitamins might be necessary if your doctor determines you're low in essentials like iron and B vitamins. The goal is to create a diet that supplies all the nutrients you need. As for antibiotics, their overuse might actually be a cause of SIBO, but when you're first being treated, you might be put on a short course to get rid of harmful bacteria. Probiotics are a divisive issue in the SIBO community, and may do more harm than good. Probiotic food, however, might be included in your diet.

What your life looks like treating SIBO

What is life like when you're treating SIBO? It can be challenging at first, but as you get better, you'll fall into routines and be able to add more foods back into your diet. Much of your cooking will be done at home where you have the most control, so equipment like a rice cooker, tea kettle, nutritional app, and more will be very useful. Since hydration is essential to proper digestion, you should always carry a water bottle with you. Other liquids like bone broth and herbal tea will also be an important part of your daily routine.

When you're treating SIBO, your life will look different than it did before. You'll be much more aware of what you're eating, *when* you're eating, and how food makes you feel.

As for "don'ts," you will no longer be snacking, eating processed foods, or eating quickly. All three of these habits are extremely-damaging to a healing digestive tract, so be very strict with yourself. If you're feeling overwhelmed and unsure about what your meals will look like now, continue to the recipe portion of this book, and you'll be comforted. Your diet can be still be varied, interesting, and delicious, as it should be.

THE BASICS OF FOLLOWING A SIBO PROGRAM

RULES AND REGULATIONS

Just like most diets out there, the dietary path to curing your SIBO will also ask you to follow a well-defined dietary guideline, which I have discussed below.

However, the dietary restrictions aren't the only rule that you should keep in mind! In fact, there are certain other lifestyle changes and restrictions that you should follow in order to further accelerate the process of healing your gut.

A quick overview of what you should keep an eye out is as follows:

- Make sure to drink as much water as possible as it is extremely crucial to your SIBO recovery. It will help your digestive system run smoothly allow you to keep your SIBO symptoms under check.

- Make sure to avoid taking antacids and proton pump inhibitors. If you lower down the amount of stomach acids by taking antacids and similar inhibitors, it will make digestion more difficult and encourage the growth of harmful bacteria in the gut as well.

- Refrain yourself from eating processed foods as they are packed to the brim with unhealthy fat, salt and sugar. These low nutrient and high fat food are extremely harmful for the gut.

- When trying to get over your SIBO, it is of paramount importance that you avoid snacking as it prevents your digestive system from getting enough time to rest and heal.

- While eating, make sure to chew your food slowly and thoroughly. It will help your body to digest foods easily and absorb the nutrients more effortlessly.

- Make sure to keep a long gap between meals, similar to what one might do during intermittent fasting. As a rule of thumb, you should have two meals a day, keeping a gap of 14 hours between dinner and breakfast next morning.

FOOD GUIDE

Like I said, the dietary restrictions are just as important as the lifestyle changes for SIBO recovery. The key is to eliminate FODMAP's from your diet. Keeping that in mind, these are the major categories that you should generally avoid:

- Polyols
- Fructans
- Galactans
- Lactose
- Fructose

Going a little bit deeper, some examples of food to avoid include:

- Peas
- Rye
- Barley
- Ice cream
- Sweetened cereals
- Dried fruit
- Apples
- Artichokes
- Cauliflower
- Garlic
- Onion
- Honey
- Agave nectar
- Soft drinks
- Asparagus

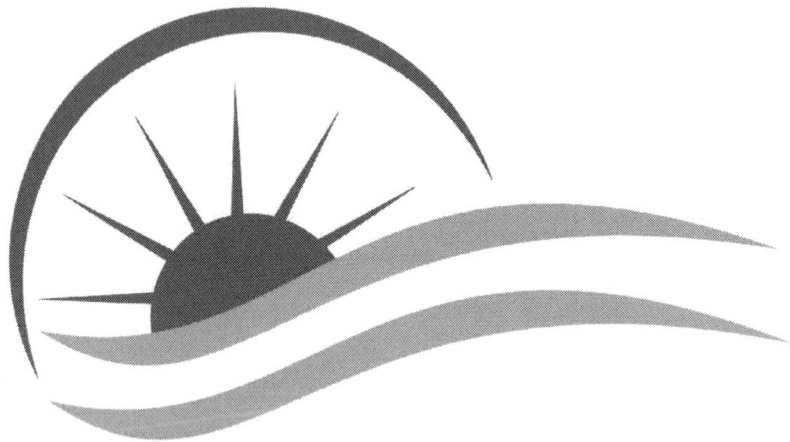

CHAPTER 1: BREAKFAST

Contents

Jalapeno Scrambled Eggs

Servings: 8 / Preparation Time: 10 minutes/ Cooking Time: 10 minutes

The perfect way to start your day! A delicious platter of spiced up scrambled eggs!

1 cup almond milk

1 tablespoon butter

6 eggs

¼ cup mushroom

Salt and pepper

- Add butter to melt into a skillet over low heat.
- Once the butter melts then add mushroom, jalapeno.
- Sauté the veggies for 5 minutes.
- Take a bowl and crack eggs into it.
- Then add almond milk and pepper into the bowl, whisk well.
- Take a skillet and pour the mixture into it.
- Cook on low heat till the eggs are fully cooked.
- Once it is ready then serve with bacon.

Per Serving: Calories: 298; Total Fat: 27g; Saturated Fat: 5g; Protein: 13g; Carbs: 1g; Fiber: 0g; Sugar: 1g

Stir-Fry Breakfast

Servings: 1 / Preparation Time: 5 minutes/ Cooking Time: 15 minutes

A simple and elegant breakfast platter to inspire you and keep you going all throughout the day!

3-4 ounces beef, grounded

1 handful veggies, chopped

1 ounce chicken liver

1 slice bacon

- Cook the bacon on low in a pan.
- In the meantime, cook the ground beef, once cooked mixed them with chicken liver.
- Add chopped veggies in the bacon.
- Strain off excess grease from ground beef mixture.
- Add baby greens.
- Serve and enjoy!

Per Serving: Calories: 475; Total Fat: 12g; Saturated Fat: 3g; Protein: 37g; Carbs: 54g; Fiber: 1g; Sugar: 8g

Kale And Avocado Skillet

Servings: 2 / Preparation Time: 5 minutes/ Cooking Time: 10 minutes

Prepare a platter full of healthy avocado and kale to start off your day with a dose of freshness!

2 tablespoons olive oil

2 cups mushrooms, sliced

5 ounces fresh kale, stemmed and sliced

1 avocado, sliced

4 large eggs

Salt and pepper to taste

- Take a large skillet and place it over medium heat.
- Add a tablespoon olive oil.
- Add mushrooms to pan and Sauté for 3 minutes.
- Take a medium bowl and massage kale with remaining 1 tablespoon olive oil (for about 1-2 minutes).
- Add kale to skillet and place them on top of mushrooms.
- Place slices of avocado on top of kale.
- Create 4 wells for eggs and crack each egg onto each hold.
- Season eggs with salt and pepper.
- Cover skillet and cook for 5 minutes.
- Serve hot!

Per Serving: Calories: 262; Total Fat: 18g; Saturated Fat: 2g; Protein: 7g; Carbs: 25g; Fiber: 1g; Sugar: 9g

Pumpkin Pancakes

Servings: 6 / Preparation Time: 5 minutes/ Cooking Time: 15 minutes

A pancake that is actually both healthy and delicious at the same time! The subtle sweet flavor coming from the pumpkin will leave you wanting more!

1 egg

3 tablespoons pumpkin puree

4 tablespoons unsweetened almond milk

A pinch of salt

1 tablespoon maple syrup

2 tablespoons oat flour

1 teaspoon pumpkin spice

½ teaspoon baking powder

- Take a bowl and add egg, almond milk, pumpkin puree, pumpkin spice, baking powder and oat flour.

- Mix them well and whisk.

- Take a pan and add oil into it.

- Heat the pan and bake pancakes for 2-3 minutes on each side and then turn them.

- Cook for 2-3 minutes.

- Drizzle with maple syrup.

- Serve and enjoy!

Per Serving: Calories: 191; Total Fat: 2g; Saturated Fat: 1g; Protein: 6g; Carbs: 45g; Fiber: 1g; Sugar: 8g

Hearty Maple Sage Breakfast

Servings: 8 / Preparation Time: 10 minutes/ Cooking Time: 20 minutes

Yet another home-style dish that incorporates the sweetness of maple and the meaty goodness of ground pork to create an energy pumping breakfast!

2 pounds ground pork

3 tablespoons finely chopped fresh sage leaves

2 tablespoons maple syrup

2 teaspoon salt

1 teaspoon pumpkin pie spice

1 teaspoon garlic oil

1 teaspoon garlic oil extra

¼ teaspoon fresh ground black pepper

1 tablespoon avocado oil

- Take a medium bowl and add pork, sage, maple syrup, salt, pumpkin pie spice, garlic oil, pepper and mix well.
- Form 6 sausage patties.
- Take a medium skillet and place it over medium-high heat, add oil and let it heat up.
- Add sausage patties and cook for 3-5 minutes per side.
- Enjoy!

Per Serving: Calories: 335; Total Fat: 26g; Saturated Fat: 5g; Protein: 19g; Carbs: 4g; Fiber: 1g; Sugar: 3g

Traditional Scrambled Eggs

Servings: 2 / Preparation Time: 10 minutes/ Cooking Time: 15 minutes

These are the most basic scrambled eggs you can get, but the addition of zucchini and spinach actually elevates the health factor up a notch.

2 tablespoons coconut oil

1 small zucchini, peeled and cut length, sliced into half moons

1 cup fresh spinach, chopped

4 large eggs, beaten

Salt and pepper as needed

¼ cup tomato, chopped

¼ avocado, chopped

2 tablespoons fresh chives, chopped

- Take a skillet and place it over medium-high heat, add oil and let it heat up.
- Add zucchini and cook for 5-10 minutes.
- Add spinach and cook for 1 minute.
- Add eggs and season with salt and pepper, cook until egg reaches your desired level of doneness.
- Divide between two serving plates, top with avocado, tomato, chives and enjoy!

Per Serving: Calories: 302; Total Fat: 26g; Saturated Fat: 4g; Protein: 14g; Carbs: 4g; Fiber: 1g; Sugar: 2g

Cheesy Omelet

Servings: 3 / Preparation Time: 10 minutes/ Cooking Time: 10 minutes

If you are tired of scrambled eggs, try out this Omelet dripping and oozing with cheese! You'll fall in love with it.

2 whole eggs

1 tablespoon water

1 tablespoon butter

5 fresh basil leaves

5 thin slices of fresh ripe tomatoes

2 ounces mozzarella cheese

Salt and pepper to taste

- Take a small bowl and whisk in eggs and water.
- Take a non-stick Sauté pan and place it over medium heat, add butter and let it melt.
- Pour egg mix and cook for 30 seconds.
- Top with cheese, tomatoes, basil slices
- Season with salt and pepper according to your taste.
- Cook for 2 minutes and fold the egg with the empty half.
- Cover and cook on LOW for 1 minute.
- Serve and enjoy!

Per Serving: Calories: 176; Total Fat: 14g; Saturated Fat: 3g; Protein: 11g; Carbs: 1g; Fiber: 1g; Sugar: 1g

Grain Free Breakfast Oatmeal

Servings: 2 / Preparation Time: 5 minutes/ Cooking Time: 5 minutes

Oatmeal is awesome when it comes to giving you a complete breakfast! But since you are on SIBO, this "Grain" free oatmeal will help you stay satisfied all throughout the day.

1 egg, beaten

4 tablespoons coconut, shredded

3 tablespoons acorn squash, cooked

½ teaspoon vanilla powder or extract

½ teaspoon honey

1 tablespoon collagen peptides

¾ cup coconut milk

1 tablespoon cinnamon

½ teaspoon sea salt

- Take a saucepan, add milk, shredded coconut and squash together into it and heat on medium heat.
- Whisk in honey, vanilla, sea salt and collagen peptides.
- Remove from the heat and rapidly whisk in the egg.
- Back to heat and cook for 2-3 minutes more.
- Drizzle with cinnamon.
- Serve with sliced banana and berries.

Per Serving: Calories: 233; Total Fat: 7g; Saturated Fat: 4g; Protein: 7g; Carbs: 38g; Fiber: 1g; Sugar: 7g

Lovely Devilled Eggs

Servings: 3 / Preparation Time: 5 minutes/ Cooking Time: 5 minutes

Nobody can say "NO" to a batch of tasty devilled eggs in the morning. If you are in a hurry, this is the dish that you need!

4 large eggs, hardboiled

2 tablespoons mayonnaise

¼ cup cheddar cheese, grated

1 jalapeno, sliced

- Cut eggs in half, remove yolk and put them in bowl.
- Lay egg whites on a platter.
- Mix in remaining ingredients and mash them with the egg yolks.
- Transfer yolk mix back to the egg whites.
- Serve and enjoy!

Per Serving: Calories: 114; Total Fat: 10g; Saturated Fat: 3g; Protein: 5g; Carbs: 1g; Fiber: 1g; Sugar: 0g

Scrambled Up Pesto Eggs

Servings: 3 / Preparation Time: 5 minutes/ Cooking Time: 5 minutes

This particular scrambled eggs recipe combines the greenish color and spiced up flavor of pesto to elevate a simple scrambled eggs recipe into something truly special.

3 large whole eggs

1 tablespoon clarified butter

1 tablespoon pesto

2 tablespoons creamed coconut milk

Salt and pepper to taste

- Take a bowl and crack open your egg.
- Season with a pinch of salt and pepper.
- Pour eggs into a pan.
- Add butter and introduce heat.
- Cook on low heat and gently add pesto.
- Once the egg is cooked and scrambled, remove heat.
- Spoon in coconut cream and mix well.
- Turn on heat and cook on LOW for a while until you have a creamy texture.
- Serve and enjoy!

Per Serving: Calories: 258; Total Fat: 10g; Saturated Fat: 3g; Protein: 14g; Carbs: 29g; Fiber: 1g; Sugar: 6g

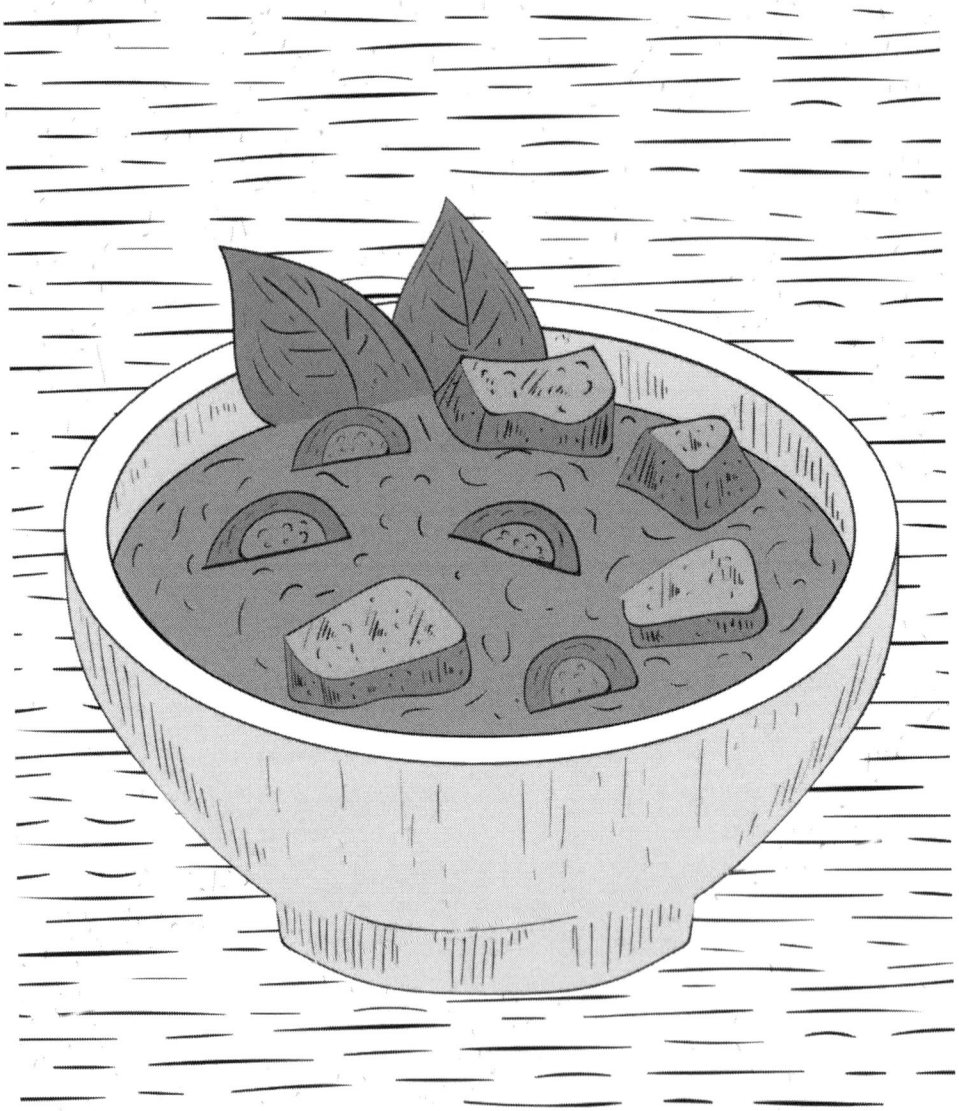

CHAPTER 2: SOUP AND SALAD

Contents

Chicken Noodles Soup

Servings: 6 / Preparation Time: 10 minutes/ Cooking Time: 15 minutes

Let me start off the soup section with the most basic soup first, a simple yet efficient chicken noodle soup for all ages.

2 cups quinoa or brown rice noodles, uncooked

2 cups chicken broth

2 tablespoons garlic-infused olive oil

4 cups water

1 teaspoon thyme

1 celery stalk, diced

3 medium carrots, sliced

½ lemon juice

2 cups chicken, cooked and diced

Parsley, optional

Salt and pepper

- Heat up oil on medium-high temperature.
- Add carrots and celery, then cook for 5 minutes,
- Stir occasionally.
- Add broth, water, thyme and noodles.
- Bring to boil, then simmer it for 10 minutes on low heat.
- Add chicken and lemon juice then cook till warm.
- Before serving add parsley, salt and pepper.
- Enjoy!

Per Serving: Calories: 196; Total Fat: 5g; Saturated Fat: 3g; Protein: 18g; Carbs: 20g; Fiber: 1g; Sugar: 5g

Perfect Detox Veggie Soup

Servings: 8 / Preparation Time: 10 minutes/ Cooking Time: 20 minutes

This carefully crafted soup is designed to easily detox your body from the toxins that may have buried themselves inside you!

2 cups zucchini, chopped

½ pound green beans

½ cup celery, chopped

2 tablespoons fresh ginger, peeled and coarsely chopped

¼ cup fresh parsley leaves

¼ cup extra fresh parsley, chopped

2 quarts water

2 tablespoons coconut oil

1 and ½ teaspoon salt

- Take a large soup pot and place it over high heat.
- Add zucchini, green beans, celery, ginger, parsley leaves, water and bring the mixture to a boil.
- Cover pot and boil for 15 minutes until beans are soft.
- Remove heat and add coconut oil and salt.
- Blend the whole mixture using an immersion blender and puree until smooth.
- Stir in chopped parsley and stir.
- Serve and enjoy!

Per Serving: Calories: 47; Total Fat: 4g; Saturated Fat: 1g; Protein: 1g; Carbs: 3g; Fiber: 1g; Sugar: 1g

_The Great Moroccan Carrot Soup

Servings: 4 / Preparation Time: 10 minutes/ Cooking Time: 30 minutes

A carrot soup that represents the brave flavor palette of Morocco, what more could you ask for?

½ cup (24 hours yogurt)

1 teaspoon ground cumin

2 tablespoons organic grass fed butter

3 scallions, dark green parts only, sliced

1 pound carrots, diced

2 and ½ cups chicken broth

1 tablespoon pasteurized clover honey

1 teaspoon fresh squeezed lemon juice

1/8 teaspoon ground allspice

- Take a small bowl and stir in yogurt, cumin.
- Take a medium soup pot and place it over medium-high heat, add butter and melt.
- Add scallions and Sauté for 2 minutes.
- Add carrots and Sauté for 4 minutes.
- Add broth and bring to a boil, lower heat to medium-low and simmer for 20 minutes.
- Use an immersion blender to puree the soup.
- Whisk in honey, lemon juice and allspice.
- Ladle soup into bowls and top with dollops of cumin yogurt, enjoy!

Per Serving: Calories: 175; Total Fat: 5g; Saturated Fat: 1g; Protein: 10g; Carbs: 19g; Fiber: 1g; Sugar: 11g

Authentic Chicken Caesar Salad

Servings: 1 / Preparation Time: 10 minutes/ Cooking Time: nil

The classical Caesar Salad re-invented to be simple and much easier to prepare!

2 cups romaine lettuce leaves, chopped

2 tablespoons Caesar Salad Dressing

1 cup organic chicken, shredded

2 tablespoons parmesan cheese, grated

1 large hardboiled egg, sliced

- Take a bowl and add lettuce, add dressing and coat all the leaves.
- Scatter chicken and sprinkle cheese all over.
- Top with sliced egg and enjoy!

Per Serving: Calories: 459; Total Fat: 25g; Saturated Fat: 5g; Protein: 40g; Carbs: 17g; Fiber: 1g; Sugar: 4g

Coconut Carrot Ginger Soup

Servings: 4 / Preparation Time: 10 minutes/ Cooking Time: 20 minutes

If you are looking for a more traditional carrot soup, then this coconut carrot and ginger soup is the one that you should go for!

4 cups vegetables stock or boiling water

4 parsnips

4 tablespoons coconut milk

1 tablespoon paprika

1 teaspoon turmeric

3 medium carrots, sliced

1 inch chunk of ginger

1 tablespoon organic apple cider vinegar

Dash of sea salt and pepper

- Peel the carrots, parsnips and ginger then chop into chunks.
- Take a large pan and put all veggies including ginger into it.
- Mix turmeric, paprika, salt and pepper together.
- Simmer for 20 minutes.
- Allow it cool then transfer everything into a blender.
- Pour in organic apple cider vinegar and coconut milk, blend till smooth.
- When serving, top with a splash of coconut milk.
- Serve and enjoy!

Per Serving: Calories: 158; Total Fat: 7g; Saturated Fat: 1g; Protein: 2g; Carbs: 23g; Fiber: 1g; Sugar: 11g

Cool Orangey Salad

Servings: 2 / Preparation Time: 10 minutes/ Cooking Time: nil

Oranges are often considered for juices, but this recipe will teach you how to prepare a feisty salad with orange!

2 cups soft organic lettuce

2 large orange, peeled and segmented

½ cup Kalamata olives, pitted and halved

2-3 tablespoons mustard vinaigrette

1 teaspoon fresh parsley, chopped

- Divide the lettuce between two small plates.
- Take a small bowl and add orange segments, olives.
- Add vinaigrette to the bowl and toss to coat well.
- Top lettuce with orange, olive mixture and sprinkle parsley.
- Enjoy!

Per Serving: Calories: 465; Total Fat: 40g; Saturated Fat: 1g; Protein: 3g; Carbs: 27g; Fiber: 1g; Sugar: 12g

Zucchini and Tomato Soup

Servings: 4 / Preparation Time: 5 minutes/ Cooking Time: 40 minutes

A perfect soup that where the tangy and bitter flavors are deliciously balanced due to the addition of zucchini and tomatoes.

2 pounds zucchini, sliced

2 tablespoons gluten free flour

8 cups vegetables stock

4 cups tomatoes, chopped

2 celery sticks, chopped

1 tablespoon olive oil

½ teaspoon turmeric

Pepper, to taste

- Take a pan and heat up over oil.
- Add zucchini and celery into the pan and cook for 5 minutes.
- Stir occasionally.
- Add flour and tomatoes, then cook for 3 minutes, stir a bit.
- Add vegetable stock and turmeric, then cover the pan.
- Simmer on low for 30 minutes.
- Puree the vegetables by using a blender.
- Sieve for added smoothness if you want.
- Serve with gluten-free bread.
- You can store it in the freezer for up to 2 months.
- Enjoy!

Per Serving: Calories: 492; Total Fat: 41g; Saturated Fat: 10g; Protein: 8g; Carbs: 24g; Fiber: 1g; Sugar: 16g

Great Zucchini Pureed Soup

Servings: 4 / Preparation Time: 5 minutes/ Cooking Time: 20 minutes

A hearty soup where zucchini steals the show!

3 tablespoons ghee

4 medium zucchini, peeled and cut lengthwise, sliced into half moons

4 cups vegetable broth

Salt and pepper as needed

- Take a medium saucepan and place it over medium-high heat, add ghee and let it melt.
- Add zucchini and Sauté for 10 minutes.
- Add broth and bring to a boil. Lower heat to medium-low and simmer for 10 minutes.
- Use immersion blender to blend until smooth.
- Season with salt and pepper and enjoy!

Per Serving: Calories: 86; Total Fat: 7g; Saturated Fat: 2g; Protein: 1g; Carbs: 8g; Fiber: 1g; Sugar: 4g

Dark Green Scallion Soup

Servings: 4 / Preparation Time: 5 minutes/ Cooking Time: 20 minutes

The original no fuss scallion soup that is sure to clear up your gut and revitalize your innards!

3 tablespoons organic grass-fed butter

1 scallion, dark green parts, chopped

1 celery stalk, chopped

5 cups stalk, chopped

6 cups chicken broth

Salt as needed

- Take a heavy-bottomed saucepan and place it over medium-high heat, add butter and let it melt.

- Add scallions and celery and cook for 8-10 minutes.

- Add broth and bring to a low boil. Lower heat to medium-low and simmer for 20-25 minutes.

- Use immersion blender to puree the whole mixture until smooth.

- Season with salt and pepper and enjoy!

Per Serving: Calories: 82; Total Fat: 7g; Saturated Fat: 2g; Protein: 1g; Carbs: 8g; Fiber: 1g; Sugar: 4g

Fresh Fruity Mint Salad

Servings: 3 / Preparation Time: 10 minutes/ Cooking Time: nil

This one's a fan favorite! A fruity salad that protrudes a very minty and hearty flavor. Yum!

¼ cup fresh lime, squeezed

¼ cup pasteurized clover honey

¼ cup fresh mint leaves, chopped

1 cup organic blueberries

1 cup organic strawberries

1 cup organic raspberries

1 cup halved organic grapes

- Take a medium bowl and whisk in lime juice, honey.
- Stir in mint.
- Add fruit to the bowl and stir well to combine, serve and enjoy!
- Add fruit to the bowl and gently stir, enjoy!

Per Serving: Calories: 127; Total Fat: 0g; Saturated Fat: 1g; Protein: 1g; Carbs: 31g; Fiber: 1g; Sugar: 25g

Easy Lettuce Salad

Servings: 6 / Preparation Time: 10 minutes/ Cooking Time: nil

If you are turtle lover and want to feel just how much turtles enjoy eating lettuce, this turtle salad is the one to go with!

2 ounces Romaine lettuce

½ ounces clarified butter

1 ounces Adam cheese, sliced

½ avocado, sliced

1 cherry tomato, sliced

- Add butter on top of each lettuce leaves.
- Add alternating layers of cheese, avocado, tomato slices.
- Serve and enjoy!

Per Serving: Calories: 53; Total Fat: 5g; Saturated Fat: 1g; Protein: 1g; Carbs: 1g; Fiber: 1g; Sugar: 1g

Creamy Mushroom Soup

Servings: 4 / Preparation Time: 5 minutes/ Cooking Time: 20 minutes

Who doesn't like a bowl of warm mushroom right? This recipe takes the basic mushroom soup recipe even further and gives it a creamy twist!

1 tablespoon olive oil

20 ounces mushrooms, sliced

2 cups vegetable broth

1 cup coconut cream

¾ teaspoon salt

¼ teaspoon black pepper

- Take a large sized pot and place it over medium heat
- Add mushrooms in olive oil and Sauté for 10-15 minutes
- Make sure to keep stirring it from time to time until browned evenly
- Add vegetable broth, coconut cream, coconut milk, black pepper and salt
- Bring it to a boil and lower down the temperature to low
- Simmer for 15 minutes
- Use an immersion blender to puree the mixture
- Enjoy!

Per Serving: Calories: 193; Total Fat: 12g; Saturated Fat: 3g; Protein: 7g; Carbs: 15g; Fiber: 1g; Sugar: 6g

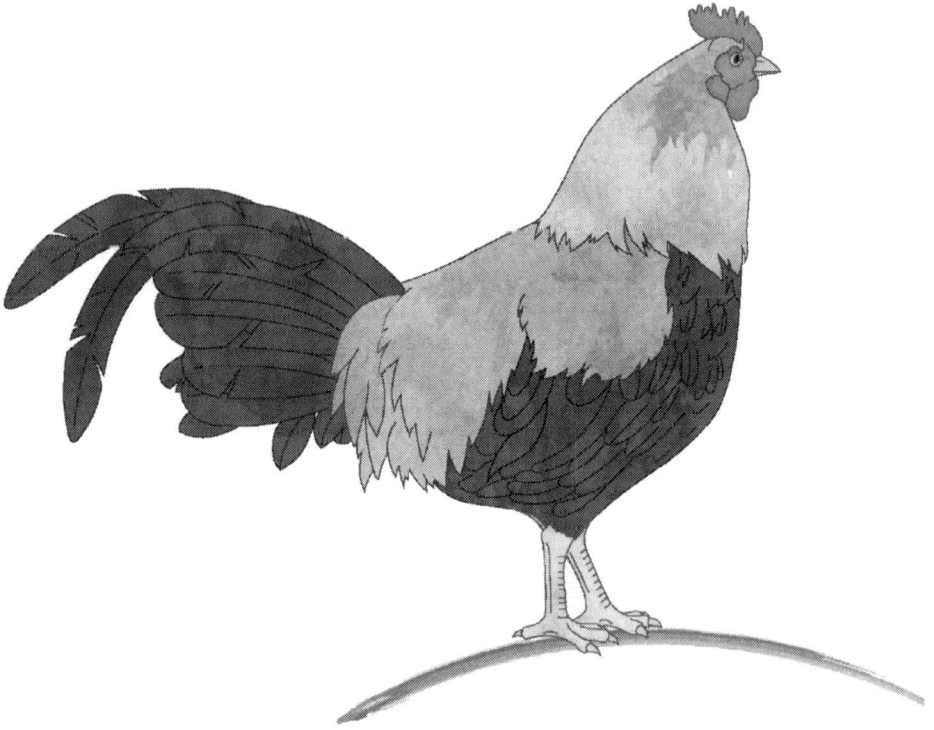

CHAPTER 3: POULTRY

Contents

Lemon Basil Chicken Dish

Servings: 8 / Preparation Time: 15 minutes/ Cooking Time: 4 minutes

Let me start off the chicken section with a very simple but amazing chicken dish that is sure to make your taste buds dance! The sour tangy taste from the lemon is to die for here!

1 tablespoon olive oil

2 tablespoons thyme, chopped

2 tablespoons oregano, chopped

10 ounces gluten free penne or fusilli

4 chicken breast, skinless

1 tablespoon white wine vinegar

1 tablespoon garlic-infused oil

3 ounces pine nuts, roasted

1 handful basil, fresh

2 ounces bag rocket

1 lemon juice

1 lemon zest

Parmesan, grated, for serving

- Preheat your oven to 390 degree F.
- Cook pasta, drain and put the side for now.
- Mix lemon zest, basil pine nuts and oil, by using mortar and pestle.
- Place chicken breast between sheets of clingy film.
- Smack the breast with a rolling pin till it becomes around 1/2" in thickness.
- Allow to heat your barbecue or griddle.
- Cook for 4 minutes on each side.
- Slice chicken, add this into the pasta with juices.
- Add rocket, basil, lemon juice and all seasoning.
- Serve and enjoy!

Per Serving: Calories: 374; Total Fat: 31g; Saturated Fat: 7g; Protein: 19g; Carbs: 5g; Fiber: 1g; Sugar: 1g

Crisp Spiced Chicken

Servings: 8 / Preparation Time: 8 minutes/ Cooking Time: 10 minutes

A very crispy but slightly spicy chicken dish that is carefully designed to help you bring a fine level of crunch to your platter!

8 chicken breast

2 tablespoons paprika

2 tablespoons turmeric

4 tablespoons coriander, ground

1 teaspoon celery salt

Black pepper, freshly grounded

4 tablespoons plain flour, gluten free

4 tablespoons cumin, ground

Sunflower oil

2 tablespoons mayonnaise

- Slice the lengthways into bite-sized pieces.
- Dust in flour and place aside.
- Take a large heavy frying pan, heat sunflower oil into it.
- Take a bowl and mix celery salt, cumin, paprika, coriander, turmeric and black pepper into it.
- Dip chicken pieces into the egg and then into the mixture of spices.
- Put chicken pieces to the pan and fry for 3-4 minutes.
- Take kitchen paper and allow it drain on it.
- Take a bowl and combine mayonnaise and coriander into the bowl.
- Serve with chicken and enjoy!

Per Serving: Calories: 248; Total Fat: 11g; Saturated Fat: 4g; Protein: 22g; Carbs: 15g; Fiber: 1g; Sugar: 10g

Lovely Bacon Wrapped Chicken Livers

Servings: 4 / Preparation Time: 10 minutes/ Cooking Time: 10 minutes

While there are some people who don't like the taste of livers, this recipe might just as easily change your perception and help you appreciate chicken livers on a whole new level!

1 pound organic chicken livers, rinsed and patted dry

½ pound bacon, halved lengthwise

Ranch dressing for dipping

- Pre-heat your oven to Broil and place a baking rack on rimmed baking sheet.
- Line with parchment paper.
- Wrap each chicken liver in piece of bacon and secure with toothpick.
- Transfer wrapped livers to prepared rack and broil for 6-8 minutes.
- Turn over and broil for 6-8 minutes more.
- Serve with ranch dressing, enjoy!

Per Serving: Calories: 485; Total Fat: 40g; Saturated Fat: 8g; Protein: 34g; Carbs: 3g; Fiber: 1g; Sugar: 0g

Chili Chicken

Servings: 4 / Preparation Time: 10 minutes/ Cooking Time: 25 minutes

If you are looking for a chicken dish that is both delicious and spicy, then this is the one to go with! You won't regret giving this dish your time.

8 boneless chicken thighs, skinless and cut into chunks

4 tablespoons vegetable oil

1 scallion, green end only, finely sliced to garnish

2 tablespoons white vinegar

Freshly steamed rice, to serve

Pinch of salt

2 red chilies

2 tablespoons fresh root ginger, finely grated

1 tablespoon garlic infused oil

2 tablespoons soy free seasoning sauce

2 tablespoons sesame seeds

- Take a large frying pan or wok, heat oil over medium heat into it.
- Add chilies and cook for 3-4 minutes until blackened.
- Stir in garlic infused oil and ginger and cook for about 10 minutes.
- Let it cover until tender completely.
- Add in chicken and cook until well cooked or for 8-10 minutes.
- Stir in seasoning sauce, salt and vinegar as much needed.
- Let it simmer for 1 minute. Then take a platter and place the chicken.
- Sprinkle over sesame seeds, scallions.
- Serve with steamed rice and enjoy!

Per Serving: Calories: 326; Total Fat: 18g; Saturated Fat: 4g; Protein: 26g; Carbs: 16g; Fiber: 1g; Sugar: 4g

Tender Poached Chicken Breast

Servings: 4 / Preparation Time: 5 minutes/ Cooking Time: 35 minutes

You have all tried poached eggs! But have you ever heard of poached chicken breasts? If this dish is completely new to you, then be prepared to be dazzled!

1 pound boneless chicken breast, skinless and organic

2 cups cold water

2 teaspoons Italian seasoning (without garlic)

2 bay leaves

1 organic lemon, sliced

- Add chicken breasts in heavy-bottomed medium saucepan, cover with water and add Italian seasoning, bay leaves, lemon slices.

- Bring the mix to a boil over high heat and lower heat to low, partially cover pan and simmer for 10 minutes.

- Remove heat and leave chicken breasts in hot poaching liquid for 20 minutes.

- Remove chicken from liquid and let it cool

- Slice/shred and enjoy!

Per Serving: Calories: 179; Total Fat: 4g; Saturated Fat: 2g; Protein: 32g; Carbs: 0g; Fiber: 1g; Sugar: 0g

Peri Peri Chicken

Servings: 6 / Preparation Time: 2 hours and 10 minutes/ Cooking Time: 15 minutes

The classical Peri-Peri chicken dish carefully modified for the SIBO diet. Perfect for any occasion and party!

2 tablespoons cayenne pepper

8 chicken thighs, skinless and boneless

¼ cup garlic-infused olive oil

1 cup fresh lemon juice

¼ cup paprika

1" minced pieces ginger

1 teaspoon salt

- Take a large bowl and whisk together cayenne, paprika, ginger, lemon juice, olive oil and salt into the bowl.
- Add in the chicken and coat it with the mixture by stirring.
- Marinate in a fridge for a minimum of 2 hours up to overnight.
- Preheat grill.
- Get the chicken from marinade and grill it while turn into halfway through.
- Serve and enjoy!

Per Serving: Calories: 208; Total Fat: 10g; Saturated Fat: 3g; Protein: 23g; Carbs: 5g; Fiber: 1g; Sugar: 2g

Baked Parmesan Chicken

Servings: 2 / Preparation Time: 5 minutes/ Cooking Time: 20 minutes

A very simple chicken dish that is jam packed with a bucket load of cheese with every bite! Yum.

2 tablespoons ghee

2 boneless chicken breasts, skinless

Pink salt

Fresh ground black pepper

½ cup mayonnaise

¼ cup parmesan cheese, grated

1 tablespoon dried Italian seasoning

¼ cup crushed pork rinds

- Pre-heat your oven to 425 degree F.
- Take a large baking dish and coat with ghee.
- Pat chicken breasts dry and wrap with towel.
- Season with salt and pepper .
- Place in baking dish.
- Take a small bowl and add mayonnaise, parmesan cheese, Italian seasoning.
- Slather mayo mix evenly over chicken breast.
- Sprinkle crushed pork rinds on top.
- Bake for 20 minutes until topping is browned.
- Serve and enjoy!

Per Serving: Calories: 495; Total Fat: 27g; Saturated Fat: 15g; Protein: 45g; Carbs: 16g; Fiber: 1g; Sugar: 1g

Almond Coated Chicken

Servings: 3 / Preparation Time: 15 minutes/ Cooking Time: 15 minutes

This chicken dish takes a slightly different route and introduces a crunchy almond layer on top of its body to give a tender inside and deliciously crispy outside!

2 large chicken breasts, boneless and skinless

1/3 cup lemon juice

1 and ½ cups seasoned almond meal

2 tablespoons coconut oil

Lemon pepper, to taste

Parsley as needed

- Slice chicken breast in half.
- Pound out each half until ¼ inch thick.
- Take a pan and place it over medium heat, add oil and heat it up.
- Dip each chicken breast slice into lemon juice and let it sit for 2 minutes.
- Turnover and the let the other side sit for 2 minutes as well.
- Transfer to almond meal and coat both sides.
- Add coated chicken to the oil and fry for 4 minutes per side, making sure to sprinkle lemon pepper liberally.
- Transfer to a paper lined sheet and repeat until all chicken are fried.
- Garnish with parsley and enjoy!

Per Serving: Calories: 197; Total Fat: 15g; Saturated Fat: 7g; Protein: 14g; Carbs: 1g; Fiber: 1g; Sugar: 1g

Black Berry Chicken Wings

Servings: 4 / Preparation Time: 35 minutes/ Cooking Time: 50 minutes

Combining berries and chicken might seem like a very weird combination at first, but once you try it, you will keep coming back for more!

3 pounds chicken wings

½ cup blackberry chipotle jam

Salt and pepper to taste

½ cup water

- Add water and jam to a bowl and mix well.
- Place chicken wings in a zip bag and add two-thirds of marinade.
- Season with salt and pepper.
- Let it marinate for 30 minutes.
- Pre-heat your oven to 400 degree F.
- Prepare a baking sheet and wire rack, place chicken wings in wire rack and bake for 15 minutes.
- Brush remaining marinade and bake for 30 minutes more.
- Enjoy!

Per Serving: Calories: 204; Total Fat: 5g; Saturated Fat: 1g; Protein: 33g; Carbs: 6g; Fiber: 1g; Sugar: 4g

Chicken And Zucchini Zoodles

Servings: 3 / Preparation Time: 10 minutes/ Cooking Time: 10 minutes

Why settle with traditional high carb noodles when you can get an even better experience with Zucchini Zoodles? And if simple Zoodles seem boring to you, just go ahead and add chicken to make a supreme dish!

2 chicken fillets, cubed

2 tablespoons ghee

1 pound tomatoes, diced

½ cup basil, chopped

¼ cup coconut milk

1 zucchini, shredded

- Sauté cubed chicken in ghee until no longer pink.
- Add tomatoes and season with salt.
- Simmer and reduce liquid.
- Prepare your zucchini Zoodles by shredding zucchini in food processor.
- Add basil, coconut milk to chicken and cook for a few minutes.
- Add half of the zucchini Zoodles to a bowl and top with creamy tomato basil chicken.
- Enjoy!

Per Serving: Calories: 218; Total Fat: 10g; Saturated Fat: 3g; Protein: 23g; Carbs: 8g; Fiber: 1g; Sugar: 5g

Super Easy Oven Baked Chicken

Servings: 4 / Preparation Time: 10 minutes/ Cooking Time: 50 minutes

The classical oven baked chicken even easier and compatible with SIBO! Just go ahead and you will thoroughly enjoy!

3 pounds skin-on organic chicken, thighs, legs or breasts

Salt and pepper to taste

1 cup white rice flour

½ teaspoon paprika

½ teaspoon Italian seasoning (no garlic)

1 tablespoon organic grass fed butter, melted

1 tablespoon garlic oil

- Pre-heat your oven to 400 degrees F.
- Line a baking sheet with parchment paper.
- Pat chicken dry with paper towels and season with salt and pepper.
- Take a gallon sized re-sealable bag and add white rice flour, paprika, Italian seasoning and seal, shake well to mix everything.
- Add half of the chicken to the bag and seal, shake well.
- Transfer chicken to prepped sheet and repeat with rest of the chicken.
- Take a small bowl and stir in butter and garlic oil. Drizzle mix over chicken.
- Bake for 50 minutes.
- Enjoy!

Per Serving: Calories: 313; Total Fat: 20g; Saturated Fat: 6g; Protein: 25g; Carbs: 9g; Fiber: 2g; Sugar: 0g

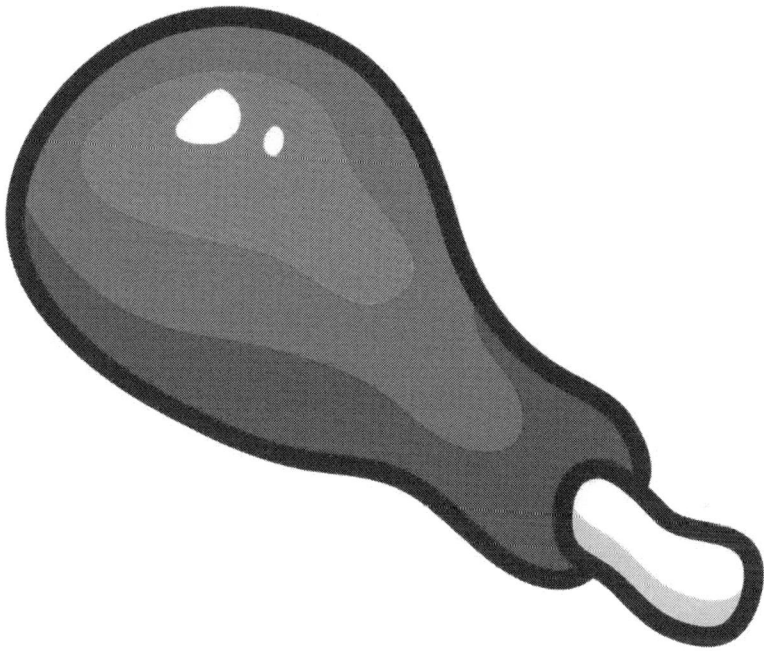

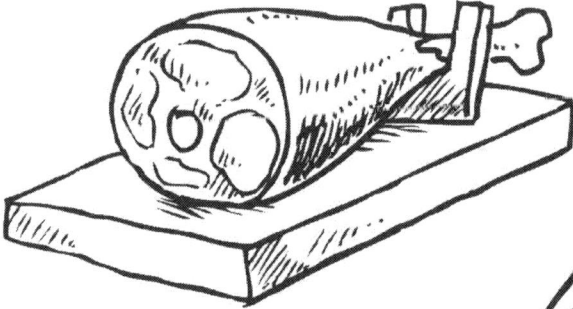

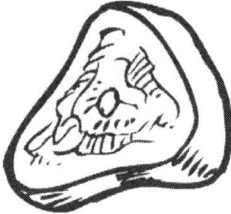

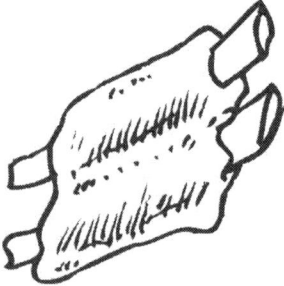

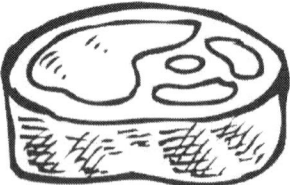

CHAPTER 4: MEAT

Contents

Pesto Turkey Meatballs

Servings: 8 / Preparation Time: 10 minutes/ Cooking Time: 30 minutes

Let's start off the meat section with a very homely and traditional turkey meatballs! And these not ordinary meatballs, these are thoroughly flavored with a gorgeous pesto sauce. Yum!

2 pounds turkey, ground

¼ cup fresh chives

½ cup fresh basil

¼ cup garlic-infused oil

1 lemon, zest and juice

- Preheat your oven to 375 degree F.
- Use aluminum foil to line a rimmed baking sheet.
- Blend basil, olive oil, chives, lemon zest and juice in a blender.
- Blend until smooth.
- Take a large bowl and mix together pesto mixture and turkey into it.
- Make balls and arrange on baking sheet.
- Bake for 25-30 minutes.
- Serve warm and enjoy!

Per Serving: Calories: 515; Total Fat: 20g; Saturated Fat: 3g; Protein: 33g; Carbs: 20g; Fiber: 1g; Sugar: 3g

Fancy Asian Ground Pork Ala Lettuce Cups

Servings: 4 / Preparation Time: 20 minutes/ Cooking Time: 20 minutes

This is a very well renowned Asian recipe that combines a very deliciously prepared ground pork mash with small lettuce cups, giving you the perfect dish with a quick munch.

1 pound ground pork

2 tablespoons garlic oil

2 carrots, finely chopped

2 teaspoons Chinese five spice powder

4 scallions, dark green parts only, chopped

2 teaspoons gluten free fish sauce

½ cup fresh cilantro, chopped

½ cup fresh Thai basil leaves, chopped

1/3 cup fresh mint leaves, chopped

1 large head butter lettuce, leaves separated

½ English cucumber, peeled, seeded and diced

1 pint organic cherry tomatoes, halved

- Take a large skillet and place it over high heat, add pork and Sauté for 5-7 minutes.
- Add garlic oil, carrots, five spice powder, scallions and cook for 5-10 minutes.
- Remove the heat and transfer to a large bowl.
- Stir in fish sauce, cilantro, basil and mint.
- Serve spoonful of the mixture in lettuce leaves, topped up with cucumber and tomatoes.
- Enjoy!

Per Serving: Calories: 151; Total Fat: 11g; Saturated Fat: 1g; Protein: 4g; Carbs: 13g; Fiber: 1g; Sugar: 55g

French Oven Beef Stew

Servings: 4 / Preparation Time: 15 minutes/ Cooking Time: 4 hours

The French are well known for their onion soup, but since SIBO doesn't allow us to have onion, let's go with the best next thing! The authentic French oven baked beef stew. Magnifique!

4 potatoes	4 cups tomatoes, chopped
¼ cup tapioca	1 celery stalk
1 pound beef	1 cup tomato juice
1 cup funnel bulb, diced	½ teaspoon turmeric
4 parsnips	Pepper, to taste

- Preheat your oven to 300 degree.
- Slice beef into 1 and ½ inch cubes.
- Wash your vegetables and dice and chop them properly.
- Take a large dish then add everything except the potatoes into it.
- Cover the dish and bake for 3 minutes.
- After that, add potatoes and then bake for 1 hour more.
- Serve and enjoy!

Per Serving: Calories: 178; Total Fat: 11g; Saturated Fat: 3g; Protein: 4g; Carbs: 19g; Fiber: 1g; Sugar: 12g

Sesame Beef

Servings: 2 / Preparation Time: 5 minutes/ Cooking Time: 3 minutes

A simple sesame tossed beef dish that you keep you and your tummy happy for days to come!

2 tablespoons maple syrup

1 and ½ pounds steak, sliced

2 tablespoons gluten free soy sauce

2 teaspoons sunflower oil

2 teaspoons sesame seeds

- Take a wok and heat up it till the oil starts to smoke.
- Add beef and stir-fry for about 2 minutes on high.
- When you start stir-frying then do not move the contents too much for first 30 seconds.
- Add sesame seeds and cook for another minute.
- After that, mix in the maple syrup.
- Toss it up and everything has to be coated well.
- Add soy sauce and cook for a few minutes.
- Allow it to bubble for a moment.
- Serve over rice and enjoy!

Per Serving: Calories: 319 Total Fat: 20g; Saturated Fat: 4g; Protein: 22g; Carbs: 13g; Fiber: 1g; Sugar: 2g

Avocado Beef Patties

Servings: 2 / Preparation Time: 15 minutes/ Cooking Time: 10 minutes

A very simple and easy to follow recipe that helps you create fancy beef patties that protrude a very nice tangy flavor from the avocados!

1 pound lean ground beef

1 small avocado, pitted and peeled

2 slices yellow cheddar cheese

Salt and pepper to taste

- Pre-heat and prepare your broiler to high.
- Divide beef into two equal sized patties.
- Season the patties with salt and pepper accordingly.
- Broil the patties for 5 minutes per side.
- Transfer the patties to a platter and add cheese.
- Slice avocado into strips and place them on top of the patties.
- Serve and enjoy!

Per Serving: Calories: 714; Total Fat: 37g; Saturated Fat: 7g; Protein: 36g; Carbs: 48g; Fiber: 1g; Sugar: 7g

Beef Sauté And Zucchini With Coriander

Servings: 2 / Preparation Time: 10 minutes/ Cooking Time: 10 minutes

Easy to make simple Beef Sauté dish that is made even wonderful thanks to the addition of Coriander and Zucchini. A healthy and beefy punch.

10 ounces beef, sliced into 1-2 inch strips

1 zucchini, cut into 2 inch strips

¼ cup parsley, chopped

2 tablespoons tamari sauce

4 tablespoons avocado oil

- Add 2 tablespoons avocado oil in a frying pan over high heat.
- Place strips of beef and brown for a few minutes on high heat.
- Once the meat is brown, add zucchini strips and Sauté until tender.
- Once tender, add tamari sauce, parsley and let them sit for a few minutes more.
- Serve immediately and enjoy!

Per Serving: Calories: 218; Total Fat: 10g; Saturated Fat: 3g; Protein: 23g; Carbs: 8g; Fiber: 1g; Sugar: 5g

Homely Lamb Chops

Servings: 4 / Preparation Time: 20 minutes/ Cooking Time: 10 minutes

Lamb chops are pretty difficult to make in general, but this recipe will give you the perfect and most homely lamb chops ever!

1 tablespoon salt

1 tablespoon fresh rosemary, chopped

2 tablespoons garlic oil

8 grass-fed organic baby lamb chops

1 tablespoon pork fat

- Take a small bowl and add salt, rosemary and garlic oil. Coat the lamb chops with the mixture and let them sit for 15 minutes.

- Take a large skillet and place it over high heat, add fat and let it melt.

- Add lamb chops and cook for 4-5 minutes on each side, for medium rare.

- Enjoy!

Per Serving: Calories: 313; Total Fat: 21g; Saturated Fat: 3g; Protein: 29g; Carbs: 0g; Fiber: 1g; Sugar: 0g

Delicious Easy Steak

Servings: 4 / Preparation Time: 5 minutes/ Cooking Time: 30 minutes

One of the prime target of this book was to give you recipes that anyone can make! Following that tradition, this recipe gives you amazing steaks to die for, that anyone can make!

1 and ½ pounds grass fed boneless sirloin   3 tablespoons ghee

Salt and pepper as needed

- Pat the steak dry with paper towels and season both sides with salt and pepper.
- Take a large skillet and place it over high heat, add 1 tablespoon ghee and let it heat up.
- Add steak and cook for 2 minutes, flip and add 2 tablespoons of ghee, cook for 2 minutes more and keep basting the steak with ghee.
- Flip and cook for 6 minutes more for a medium-rare meat.
- Transfer to cutting board and wrap loosely with aluminum foil.
- Let it rest for 10 minutes and cut against grain, enjoy!

Per Serving: Calories: 311; Total Fat: 17g; Saturated Fat: 2g; Protein: 39g; Carbs: 0g; Fiber: 1g; Sugar: 0g

Slowly Cooked Lamb Curry

Servings: 4 / Preparation Time: 15 minutes/ Cooking Time: 8 hours

This is the only recipe in the book that would require a Slow Cooker. But trust me on this one, if you are actually able to pull this off, the level of juiciness and satisfaction that you will get will be nothing short of heavenly.

2 tablespoons coconut oil

3 pounds lamb stew meat

1 (14 ounces) can full fat coconut milk

1 and ½ tablespoons fresh ginger, peeled and grated

1 tablespoon garlic oil

1 tablespoon paprika

2 teaspoons ground coriander

2 teaspoons ground cumin

1 teaspoon ground turmeric

1 (14 ounces) organic tomatoes, diced and undrained

1 and ½ teaspoons salt

- Take a large skillet and place it over high heat, add coconut oil and let it melt.
- Add stew meat in pan and brown the outside.
- Transfer each meat to your Slow Cooker once browned. Repeat until all meats are used up.
- Add coconut milk, ginger, garlic oil, coriander, paprika, cumin, turmeric, tomatoes to the Slow Cooker.
- Close lid and cook for 8 hours on LOW.
- Stir in salt and enjoy!

Per Serving: Calories: 371; Total Fat: 23g; Saturated Fat: 5g; Protein: 36g; Carbs: 5g; Fiber: 1g; Sugar: 2g

Hearty Pork Chops With Chimichurri

Servings: 2 / Preparation Time: 5 minutes/ Cooking Time: 25 minutes

We all love pork chops right? But why just have boring old regular pork chops when we can just as easily improve the flavors even more? Add a Chimicchuri sauce to the mix to completely alter your perception of Pork Chops.

2 (5 ounces each), bone in pork chops

4 teaspoons melted ghee

Salt and pepper to taste

4 tablespoons Chimichurri sauce

- Pre-heat your oven to 400 degrees F.
- Take an oven safe-skillet and place it over high heat, pat pork chops dry with paper towel and rub each with 2 teaspoons of ghee.
- Sprinkle salt and pepper all over.
- Transfer chops to pan and sear for 2 minutes on each side.
- Transfer the skillet to oven and cook for 15 minutes.
- Let the chops rest for 5 minutes and top each with 2 tablespoons of Chimichurri sauce.
- Enjoy!

Per Serving: Calories: 361; Total Fat: 0g; Saturated Fat: 0g; Protein: 40g; Carbs: 0g; Fiber: 1g; Sugar: 0g

Pork Rinds In Stick

Servings: 2 / Preparation Time: 5 minutes/ Cooking Time: 25 minutes

A very quick and easy to make dish that you can use as both a snack and even dinner dish. A perfect pork dish busy individuals.

2 medium zucchini, halved lengthwise, seeded

¼ cup pork rinds, crushed

¼ cup parmesan cheese, grated

2 tablespoons melted butter

Salt and pepper to taste

Olive oil for drizzle

- Pre-heat your oven to 400 degree F.
- Line a baking sheet with aluminum foil.
- Place zucchini halves (cut side facing up) on prepared baking sheet.
- Take a medium bowl and add pork rinds, parmesan cheese, melted butter, season with pepper and salt.
- Mix well.
- Spoon pork rind mix onto zucchini stick.
- Drizzle olive oil.
- Bake for 20 minutes until the topping is golden brown.
- Turn your broiler and brown for 3-5 minutes.
- Serve and enjoy!

Per Serving: Calories: 173; Total Fat: 5g; Saturated Fat: 2g; Protein: 7g; Carbs: 27g; Fiber: 2g; Sugar: 24g

_Mushroom Pork Chops

Servings: 3 / Preparation Time: 10 minutes/ Cooking Time: 40 minutes

Yet another pork chops dish whose flavor is further made magical thanks to the addition of finely cooked mushrooms.

8 ounces mushrooms, sliced

1 cup mayonnaise

3 pork chops, boneless

1 teaspoon ground nutmeg

1 tablespoon balsamic vinegar

½ cup coconut oil

- Take a pan and place it over medium heat.
- Add oil and let it heat up.
- Add mushrooms and stir.
- Cook for 4 minutes.
- Add pork chops, season with nutmeg, and brown both sides.
- Transfer the pan in oven and bake for 30 minutes at 350 degree F.
- Transfer pork chops to plates and keep it warm.
- Take a pan and place it over medium-heat.
- Add vinegar, mayonnaise over mushroom mix and stir or a few minutes.
- Drizzle sauce over pork chops.
- Enjoy!

Per Serving: Calories: 435; Total Fat: 28g; Saturated Fat: 6g; Protein: 42g; Carbs: 1g; Fiber: 0g; Sugar: 0g

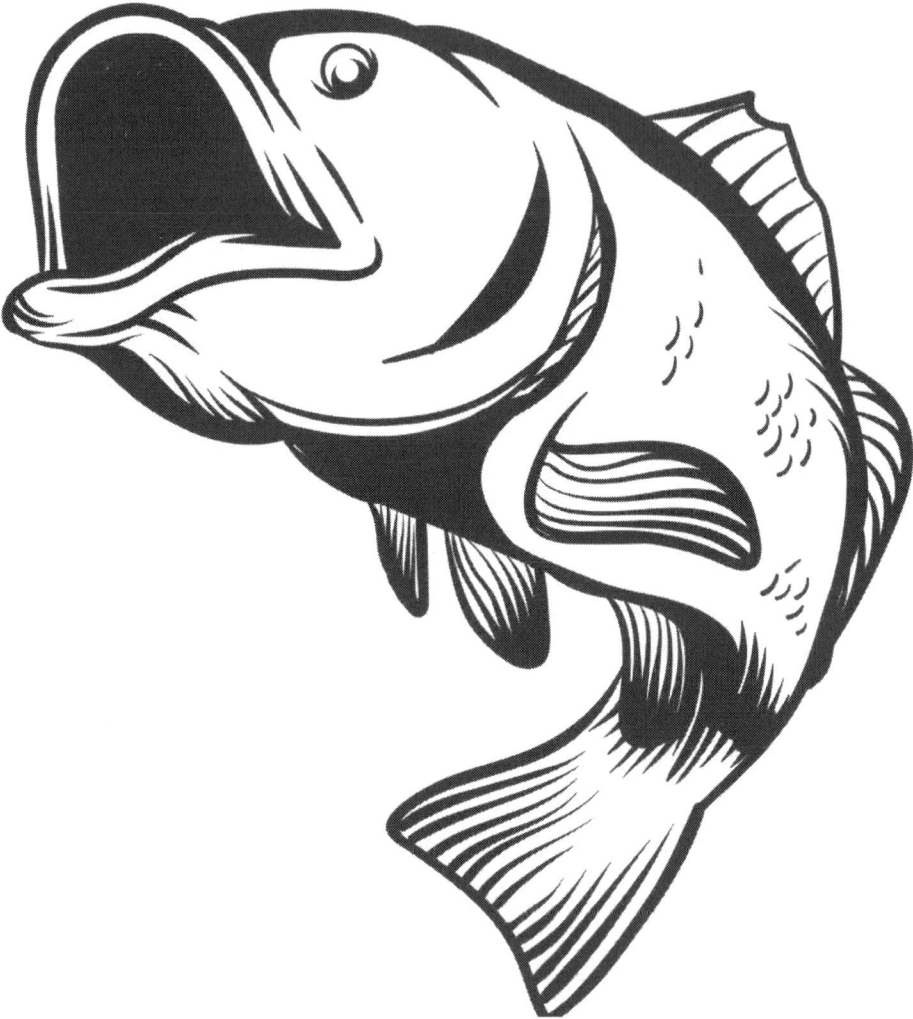

CHAPTER 5: SEAFOOD

Contents

Eat Butter with Avocado and Smoked Salmon

Servings: 2 / Preparation Time: 5 minutes/ Cooking Time: 15 minutes

Simple yet efficient, Smoke Salmon dish dredged with a hearty dose of SIBO friendly Avocado butter.

4 eggs	5 ounces clarified butter
2 tablespoons olive oil	4 ounces salmon, smoked
¼ teaspoon black pepper, grounded	2 avocado
1 tablespoon fresh parsley, chopped	½ teaspoon sea salt

- Take a pot and put the eggs and boil them with no lid.
- Simmer for 7-8 minutes on low heat.
- Take a bowl with cold water and transfer the eggs
- Peel the eggs and chop them finely.
- By using a fork, mix butter and eggs and then season with pepper and salt.
- Serve with chopped parsley.

Per Serving: Calories: 222; Total Fat: 15g; Saturated Fat: 3g; Protein: 5g; Carbs: 14g; Fiber: 1g; Sugar: 1g

Salmon Lemon Fish Cakes

Servings: 6 / Preparation Time: 5 minutes/ Cooking Time: 40 minutes

A very kid-friendly dish lemony Salmon Fish cakes dish!

2 large baking potatoes

5 ounces smoked salmon trimmings, plus extra to serve

2 tablespoons gluten-free flour mixed with 1 teaspoon grounded pepper

2 tablespoons olive oil

½ lemon juice and zest, grated

1 egg yolk

1 tablespoon frying oil

1 tablespoon parsley, chopped

- Microwave potatoes for about 10 minutes on high till soft.
- Allow to cool for 5 minutes.
- Take a bowl and scoop flesh and mash into it, allow it to cool.
- Season with olive oil, lemon juice and zest and mix in salmon, egg and parsley.
- Form small rounds on 3cm diameter and 1 cm deep and chill for about 14-25 minutes.
- Use peppered flour to dust each cake and then fry in little oil over low heat for 2-3 minutes on each side.
- Pour on kitchen paper.
- Serve with garnished salmon and parsley.

Per Serving: Calories: 519; Total Fat: 18g; Saturated Fat: 4g; Protein: 37g; Carbs: 54g; Fiber: 1g; Sugar: 9g

Lemony Shrimp Rice

Servings: 6 / Preparation Time: 5 minutes/ Cooking Time: 15 minutes

Fancy for some heavy rice meal? Try out this gorgeous Shrimp rice and be prepared to bask in its awesome flavors!

1 tablespoon olive oil

½ pound long grain rice

1 red chili

1 tablespoon chives, chopped

4 tablespoons butter, lactose free

1 teaspoon garlic oil

Juice and zest, 1 lemon

½ pound raw shrimp, peeled, defrosted if frozen

- Boil the kettle over high heat.
- Take a pan and heat oil into it with a lid.
- Add chili and fry for 3 minutes.
- Stir in rice to coat it.
- Add ½ liter of boiling water and cook for about 12 minutes when covered.
- Then uncover the pan and stir.
- In a frying pan, heat oil till hot and add shrimp.
- When it turns into pink, add butter, lemon juice and zest, chives and cook for 1 more minute.
- Cook it till rice is tender and shrimp are soft.
- Serve with rice and top with butter, shrimp and lemon.

Per Serving: Calories: 344; Total Fat: 5g; Saturated Fat: 1g; Protein: 19g; Carbs: 44g; Fiber: 1g; Sugar: 0g

Salmon And Spinach Bake

Servings: 4 / Preparation Time: 7 minutes/ Cooking Time: 15 minutes

Easy yet satisfyingly baked Salmon and Spinach delight! Perfect for quick bite.

3.5 ounces baby spinach leaves

8 ounces tub cream, lactose free

2 tablespoons wholegrain mustard

26 ounces medium potatoes, cut into wedges

2 large salmon fillets, cut into pieces

3 ounces cheddar, grated

Handful parmesan, grated

- Take a microwave-proof baking dish.
- Cook potato wedges on high for 10 minutes into the dish.
- Heat the grill to medium.
- Add mustard and lactose free cream and mix them together.
- Nestle spinach and salmon into the potatoes.
- Spoon the cream mix over to cover most spinach.
- Drizzle with cheeses and grill for more 5 minutes.
- Cook until potatoes tips turn into golden and salmon is cooked properly.
- Serve and enjoy!

Per Serving: Calories: 173; Total Fat: 11g; Saturated Fat: 3g; Protein: 14g; Carbs: 4g; Fiber: 1g; Sugar: 2g

Simple Baked White Fish

Servings: 4 / Preparation Time: 40 minutes/ Cooking Time: 20 minutes

The majestically prepared White Fish at your service! The olive oil and lemon wedges makes this one of the tastiest and healthiest fish dish around!

2-3 pounds cod

Salt as needed

¼ cup extra virgin olive oil

4 lemon wedges

1 teaspoon fresh parsley, chopped

- Rinse fish thoroughly and pat them dry with paper towels, transfer to baking pan.
- Sprinkle salt and olive oil, let them marinate for 30 minutes.
- Pre-heat your oven to 350 degrees F.
- Bake the fish for 15-20 minutes until the fish is tender.
- Squeeze lemon over fish and sprinkle parsley, serve and enjoy!

Per Serving: Calories: 309; Total Fat: 15g; Saturated Fat: 5g; Protein: 43g; Carbs: 1g; Fiber: 1g; Sugar: 0g

Awesome Mahi-Mahi And Avocado Lime

Servings: 4 / Preparation Time: 10 minutes/ Cooking Time: 10 minutes

Mahi-Mahi's aren't extremely common, and even when you are able to get your hands on one, making them might be somewhat of a hassle. This recipe tries to break this tradition though and teaches you how to prepare a very easy and awesome Mahi Mahi!

¼ cup salted ghee

2 tablespoons fresh cilantro leaves, minced

½ small avocado, ripe

1 tablespoon fresh squeezed lime juice

4 mahi-mahi fillets

Salt and pepper to taste

Paprika to taste

1 tablespoon coconut oil

- Take your food processor and add ghee, cilantro, avocado and lime juice.
- Process until smooth and transfer to a small bowl.
- Pat fish dry with paper towels and season with salt, pepper and paprika.
- Take a skillet and place it over medium-high heat, add coconut oil and let it melt.
- Add fillets and cook for 4-5 minutes, divide fish amongst four plates and top each fillet with avocado lime butter.
- Enjoy!

Per Serving: Calories: 267; Total Fat: 20g; Saturated Fat: 2g; Protein: 21g; Carbs: 1g; Fiber: 1g; Sugar: 0g

Herb-Crusted Fish

Servings: 8 / Preparation Time: 10 minutes/ Cooking Time: 13 minutes

Not all fish dishes have to be soft and tender right? This particular dish is coated with crunchy fish that gives you a fine crispy crunch after every bite.

7 ounces flat leaf parsley, chopped

2 pounds white fish, skinless

3.5 ounces snipped chives

14 ounces cold lactose free butter, diced

12 ounces bread, gluten free

4 tablespoons butter, lactose free

5 tablespoons sunflower oil

5 lemon zest

Sea salt

Pepper, freshly ground

- Preheat your oven to 400 degree F.
- Break the bread into chunks and process to coarse breadcrumbs using a blender.
- Add chives, parsley, butter and lemon zest and blend properly.
- Add pepper and salt to season.
- Take a large roasting tin and place the fish fillets into it.
- Move over the breadcrumb to mix.
- Bake fish for 8-10 minutes.
- Serve with mashed potatoes.

Per Serving: Calories: 178; Total Fat: 3g; Saturated Fat: 1g; Protein: 31g; Carbs: 6g; Fiber: 1g; Sugar: 3g

Baked Salmon with Potatoes

Servings: 2 / Preparation Time: 10 minutes/ Cooking Time: 30 minutes

A hearty baked salmon dish that will remind you of your country side!

2 salmon fillets, boneless and skinless

1 lemon, wedged

2 small baking potatoes, sliced

1 cup lactose free cream

- Preheat your oven to 180 degree F.
- Toss potatoes with olive oil.
- Take a roasting dish and arrange them.
- Season and bake in the oven for about 15 minutes.
- Turn over the potatoes and top with cream and then salmon.
- Season and further roast for 15 minutes more.
- Serve with lemon wedges and enjoy!

Per Serving: Calories: 272; Total Fat: 10g; Saturated Fat: 6g; Protein: 10g; Carbs: 36g; Fiber: 1g; Sugar: 2g

Great Tomato And Garlic Shrimp

Servings: 4 / Preparation Time: 25 minutes/ Cooking Time: 5 minutes

SIBO friendly tomato and garlic shrimp, what more could you ask for?

¼ cup extra virgin olive oil

¼ cup garlic oil

1 lemon, zest and juiced

1 tablespoon Dijon mustard (without garlic)

1/3 cup fresh parsley leaves, chopped

¼ cup fresh basil leaves, chopped

2 tablespoons chives, chopped

1 pint organic cherry tomatoes, halved

1 pound shrimp, peeled and deveined

Salt and pepper as needed

- Take a large sized bowl and add olive oil, garlic oil, lemon zest, lemon juice, mustard, ¼ cup parsley, basil and chives.

- Mix well, add tomatoes and shrimp, stir well to coat.

- Transfer bowl to fridge and chill for 15 minutes.

- Heat up large sized skillet and place it over medium-high heat.

- Add shrimp mixture and Sauté for 5 minutes until shrimps are cooked thoroughly.

- Top with remaining 1 tablespoon parsley, serve enjoy!

Per Serving: Calories: 340; Total Fat: 29g; Saturated Fat: 3g; Protein: 16g; Carbs: 6g; Fiber: 1g; Sugar: 0g

Salmon with Green Bean Salad

Servings: 3 / Preparation Time: 5 minutes/ Cooking Time: 10 minutes

A generous platter of salmon and Green Beans, a healthy treat for all ages!

2 salmon fillets, skinless

½ lemon juice and zest

1 tablespoon olive oil

½ pound green beans, trimmed

For sauce: 1 lemon, zest and juice

1 teaspoon chives, chopped

1 teaspoon dill, chopped

1 cup lactose free cream

2 glasses white wine, dry

1 teaspoon parsley, chopped

- Take a frying pan and heat olive oil over medium heat.
- Add salmon fillets and cook on each side for 3 minutes.
- Remove from pan and add in white wine and boil.
- Add cream, herbs, lemon zest and juice to the pan and make sauce by bubbling for 1 minute.
- In the meantime, boil green beans for 4-5 minutes.
- Serve beans with salmon on top and top with the sauce.
- Enjoy!

Per Serving: Calories: 349; Total Fat: 22g; Saturated Fat: 3g; Protein: 24g; Carbs: 14g; Fiber: 2g; Sugar: 6g

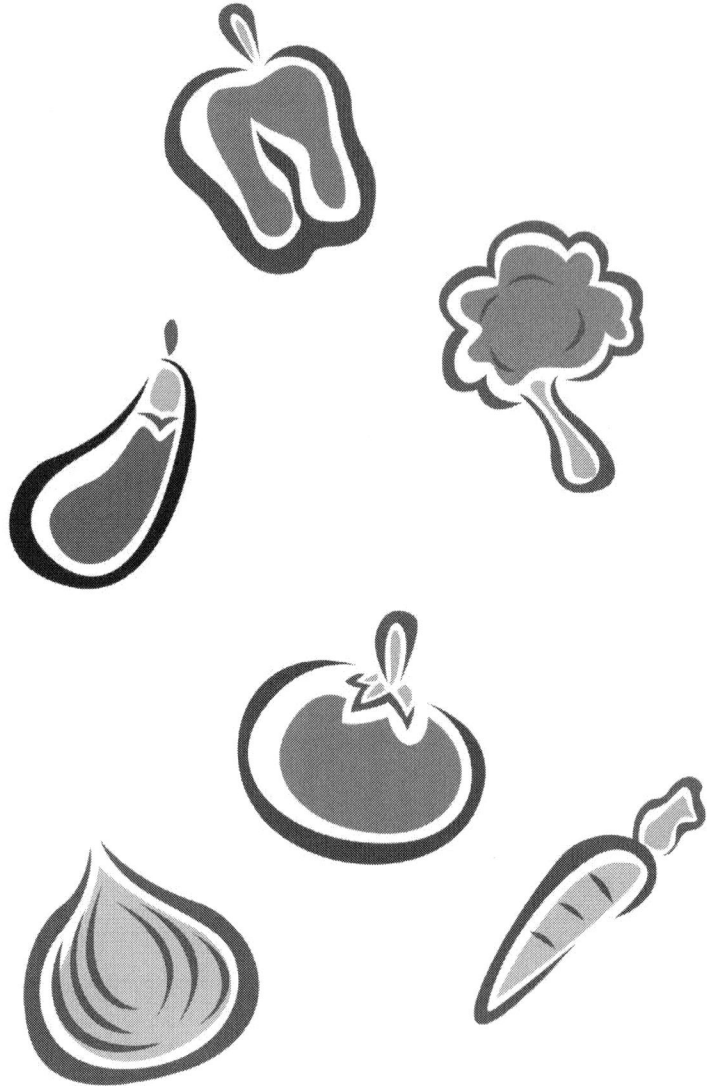

CHAPTER 6: VEGETARIAN

Contents

Sweet Roasted Maple Parsnips

Servings: 6 / Preparation Time: 10 minutes/ Cooking Time: 35 minutes

Carefully roasted Maple flavored parsnips, the perfect treat for a sweet loving vegetarian.

6 tablespoons maple syrup

8 medium parsnips

4 ounces vegetable oil

- Preheat your oven to 400 degree F.
- Wash, clean and peel parsnips.
- Cut each parsnip into four lengthwise pieces.
- Take a medium bowl and mix the parsnips with the vegetable oil into it.
- Mix with the maple syrup.
- Bake for 35 minutes.
- Serve and enjoy!

Per Serving: Calories: 259; Total Fat: 15g; Saturated Fat: 4g; Protein: 2g; Carbs: 31g; Fiber: 1g; Sugar: 14g

_Cool Hearty Baked Eggplant

Servings: 2 / Preparation Time: 10 minutes/ Cooking Time: 30 minutes

Is it a plant? Is it an egg? No! It's both, it's one of the most satisfying vegetable out there, the eggplant!

2 small eggplants, halved lengthwise

3 tablespoons fresh parsley, chopped

3 tablespoons garlic oil

Salt and pepper to taste

- Pre-heat your oven to 350 degrees F.
- Line a rimmed baking sheet with parchment paper.
- Take a sharp knife and make horizontal and vertical cuts about two thirds into the eggplant halves, forming a check board texture.
- Insert parsley into the cuts and transfer halves into the baking sheet.
- Drizzle garlic oil over eggplant and season with salt and pepper.
- Bake for 30 minutes until eggplants are tender.
- Serve and enjoy!

Per Serving: Calories: 297; Total Fat: 22g; Saturated Fat: 5g; Protein: 5g; Carbs: 27g; Fiber: 1g; Sugar: 16g

All-Time Favorite Zucchini Chips

Servings: 4 / Preparation Time: 10 minutes/ Cooking Time: 2-3 hours

You can never say no to a healthy platter of zucchini chips! Amazing for a quick bite and even better for as side dish.

4 cups thinly sliced zucchini

2 teaspoons coarse salt

2 tablespoons coconut oil, melted

- Pre-heat your oven to 200 degrees F.
- Line a baking sheet with parchment paper.
- Take a large bowl and add zucchini, coconut oil and toss well to coat them.
- Season with salt and bake for 2-3 hours until chips are crispy.
- Let the chips cool and serve, enjoy!

Per Serving: Calories: 85; Total Fat: 7g; Saturated Fat: 1g; Protein: 2g; Carbs: 5g; Fiber: 0g; Sugar: 2g

Healthy Broccoli And Lemon Butter

Servings: 4 / Preparation Time: 10 minutes/ Cooking Time: 30 minutes

Even if you hate broccoli, the lemon butter of this recipe will make your fall for them once again! Your kids will start loving them too.

1 tablespoon ghee

1 large broccoli heat, cut into bite sized portions

6 tablespoons organic grass fed butter

2 tablespoons fresh squeezed lemon juice

2 tablespoons Dijon mustard

1 teaspoon lemon zest

- Pre-heat your oven to 400 degrees F.

- Grease baking sheet with ghee and arrange broccoli in single layer.

- Season with salt and roast broccoli for 15 minutes.

- Take a small saucepan and place it over medium heat and add butter, let it melt.

- Whisk in lemon juice, mustard and lemon zest.

- Remove broccoli from oven and spoon the lemon-mustard mixture over the broccoli, bake for 10-15 minutes more.

- Serve and enjoy!

Per Serving: Calories: 278; Total Fat: 28g; Saturated Fat: 2g; Protein: 2g; Carbs: 4g; Fiber: 0g; Sugar: 1g

Brussels Platter

Servings: 3 / Preparation Time: 5 minutes/ Cooking Time: 10-15 minutes

Brussels are extremely common vegetable amongst veggie lovers! This recipe teaches you how to prepare them, the SIBO way!

¼ cup parmesan cheese

¼ cup hazelnuts, whole and skinless

1 tablespoon olive oil

1 pound Brussels sprouts

Salt to taste

- Pre-heat your oven 350 degree F.
- Line a baking sheet with parchment paper and trim bottom of Brussels.
- Put leaves in a medium sized bowl, making sure that they are broken.
- Toss leaves with olive oil and season with salt.
- Spread leaves on baking sheet.
- Roast for 10-15 minutes until crispy.
- Divide between bowls and toss with remaining ingredients.
- Serve and enjoy!

Per Serving: Calories: 107; Total Fat: 1g; Saturated Fat: 1g; Protein: 8g; Carbs: 22g; Fiber: 1g; Sugar: 6g

_Leeks Platter

Servings: 4 / Preparation Time: 10 minutes/ Cooking Time: 25 minutes

These are not the leaks in your boat! Rather, these are the leeks that your vegetarian heart craves! A butter up leek platter that will keep you coming back for more.

1 and ½ pounds leeks, trimmed and chopped into 4 inch pieces

2 ounces clarified butter

1 cup coconut cream

3 and ½ ounces cheddar cheese

Salt and pepper to taste

- Pre-heat your oven to 400 degree F.
- Take a skillet and place it over medium heat, add butter and let it heat up.
- Add leeks and Sauté for 5 minutes.
- Spread leeks in greased baking dish.
- Boil cream in saucepan and lower heat to low.
- Stir in cheese, salt and pepper.
- Pour sauce over leeks.
- Bake for 15-20 minutes and serve warm.
- Enjoy!

Per Serving: Calories: 137; Total Fat: 1g; Saturated Fat: 0g; Protein: 3g; Carbs: 32g; Fiber: 1g; Sugar: 9g

Zucchini BBQ

Servings: 4 / Preparation Time: 10 minutes/ Cooking Time: 60 minutes

Just because you like to stay on the vegetarian path, doesn't mean that you have to get rid of BBQs right? This dish will give you the perfect Zucchini BBQ ever!

Olive oil as needed

3 zucchinis

½ teaspoon black pepper

½ teaspoon mustard, garlic free

½ teaspoon cumin

1 teaspoon paprika

1 teaspoon salt

1 tablespoon chili powder

- Pre-heat your oven to 300 degree F.
- Take a small bowl and add cayenne, black pepper, salt, mustard, paprika, chili powder.
- Mix well.
- Slice zucchini into 1/8 inch slices and mist them with olive oil.
- Sprinkle spice blend over zucchini and bake for 40 minutes.
- Remove and flip, mist with more olive oil and leftover spice.
- Bake for 20 minutes more.
- Serve!

Per Serving: Calories: 479; Total Fat: 9g; Saturated Fat: 3g; Protein: 37g; Carbs: 64g; Fiber: 1g; Sugar: 24g

Simple Delight Bruschetta

Servings: 2 / Preparation Time: 5 minutes/ Cooking Time: 5 minutes

The traditional Russian Bruschetta, made in the SIBO way!

1 roasted red pepper

¼ cup feta cheese

SIBO friendly bread

1 teaspoon basil, chopped

2 tablespoons black olives, chopped

2 tomatoes, chopped

- Dice roasted red pepper.
- Mix red pepper with cheese, basil, tomatoes and olives.
- Take a medium pan and toast bread into it.
- Toast it until it turns into golden brown.
- Take a plate and place the toast.
- Serve with mixture and enjoy!

Per Serving: Calories: 283; Total Fat: 10g; Saturated Fat: 3g; Protein: 17g; Carbs: 3g; Fiber: 1g; Sugar: 1g

Warm Swiss Chard

Servings: 4 / Preparation Time: 10 minutes/ Cooking Time: 35 minutes

Very homely Swiss Chard dish that will give you a very hearty sensation after every meal.

2 tablespoons coconut oil

2 bunch Swiss chard, ribs separated and coarsely chopped

1 and ½ teaspoons garlic oil

Salt and pepper to taste

- Take a large skillet and place it over medium-high heat.

- Melt coconut oil and let it heat up.

- Add chard ribs to the skillet and Sauté for 5 minutes.

- Add chard leaves and cover skillet, lower heat to medium and cook for 10-15 minutes.

- Add garlic oil, season with salt and pepper.

- Lower heat to low and cook for 10 minutes.

- Serve and enjoy!

Per Serving: Calories: 195; Total Fat: 18g; Saturated Fat: 2g; Protein: 5g; Carbs: 10g; Fiber: 1g; Sugar: 5g

_Original Carrot Puree

Servings: 4 / Preparation Time: 5 minutes/ Cooking Time: 20 minutes

Simply put, The best carrot puree you will ever taste!

4 cups carrots, peeled and chopped

3 tablespoons coconut oil

1 tablespoon fresh ginger, peeled and chopped

Salt and pepper to taste

- Steam your carrots for 20 minutes until tender.
- Transfer to food processor and add coconut oil, ginger.
- Blend until pureed.
- Season with salt and pepper.
- Serve and enjoy!

Per Serving: Calories: 162; Total Fat: 11g; Saturated Fat: 4g; Protein: 2g; Carbs: 16g; Fiber: 1g; Sugar: 10g

All Time Favorite Spinach Sautee

Servings: 2 / Preparation Time: 5 minutes/ Cooking Time: 5 minutes

If you want to have your spinach in a very simple yet tasty way, this simple Sauté should patch your hunger up!

1 tablespoon ghee   Salt and pepper to taste

1-2 cups fresh spinach

- Take a medium skillet and place it over high heat, add ghee and let it heat up.

- Once hot, add spinach and Sauté for 2 minutes until wilted and soft.

- Season with salt and pepper.

- Serve and enjoy!

Per Serving: Calories: 149; Total Fat: 15g; Saturated Fat: 6g; Protein: 2g; Carbs: 2g; Fiber: 1g; Sugar: 0g

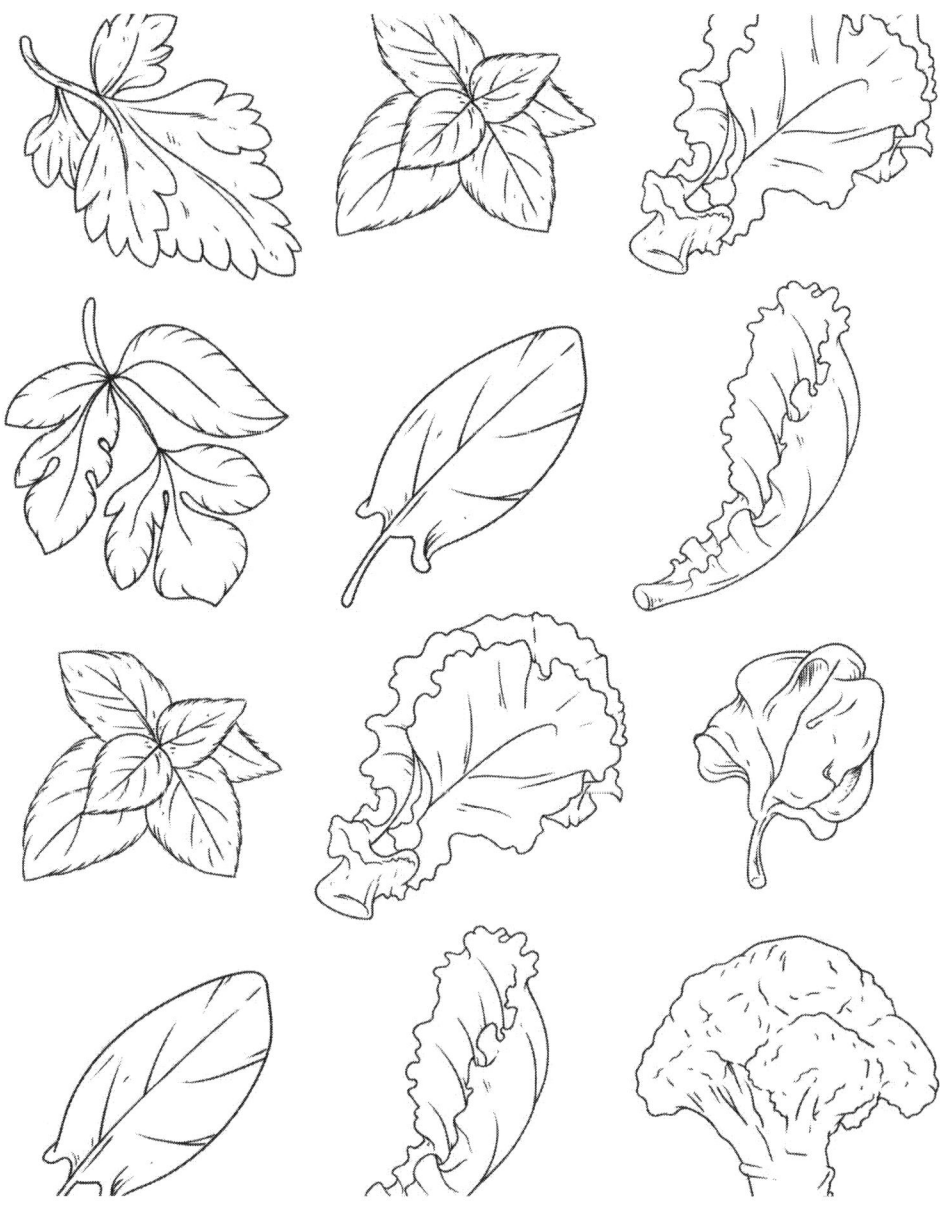

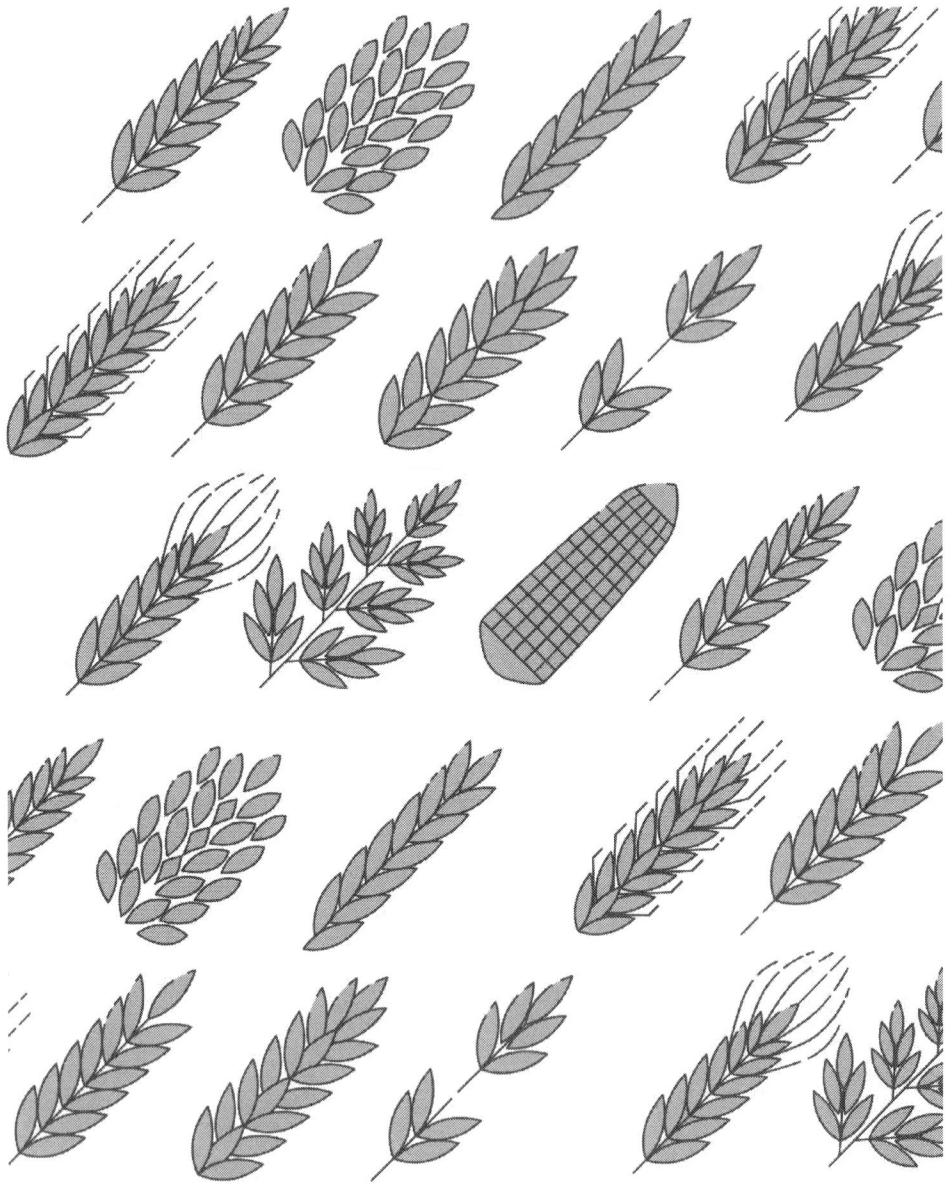

CHAPTER 7: POTATO AND GRAINS

Contents

Parmesan Herb Rice

Servings: 5 / Preparation Time: 10 minutes/ Cooking Time: 25 minutes

A herbed up parmesan rice that will go perfectly with any of your vegetarian main dish!

1 tablespoon olive oil

1 tablespoon Italian herb seasoning

¼ teaspoon black pepper, grounded

¼ cup parmesan cheese, grated

2 cups chicken broth

1 cup long grain white rice

½ teaspoon salt

- Take a large saucepan and heat olive oil over medium heat into it.
- Add rice and sauté till it is lightly brown.
- Add chicken broth, Italian herbs, salt and pepper.
- Let it boil in low heat and cover it.
- Simmer it for 15-20 minutes.
- Add in parmesan cheese and stir.
- Serve and enjoy!

Per Serving: Calories: 434; Total Fat: 13g; Saturated Fat: 3g; Protein: 13g; Carbs: 51g; Fiber: 1g; Sugar: 3g

Dill And Potato Delight

Servings: 10 / Preparation Time: 15 minutes/ Cooking Time: 20 minutes

If you are bored of simple potato recipes, this mustard-y potato dish with some dill spread around should satisfy your potato lust perfectly!

2 tablespoons Dijon mustard

¼ cup chives, minced

2 pounds red potatoes

1 lemon juice and zest

¼ cup garlic-infused olive oil

1 tablespoon vinegar

¼ cup fresh dill, chopped

Salt and pepper

- Boil water in a large pot. Add potatoes and cook for 15 minutes.
- Drain water, let it cool down then cut into quarters and set to the side.
- Whisk dill, chives, vinegar, olive oil, lemon juice and zest and mustard.
- Pour that on potatoes and then stir all together till potatoes are coated fully.
- Add salt and pepper.
- Serve and store rest in refrigerator.

Per Serving: Calories: 266; Total Fat: 12g; Saturated Fat: 7g; Protein: 5g; Carbs: 37g; Fiber: 1g; Sugar: 3g

Tender Sweet Potato Hash

Servings: 4 / Preparation Time: 10 minutes/ Cooking Time: 40 minutes

On the topic of potatoes, we should not let go of potato hash right? Just try this one out, you'll love it!

2 cups cubed sweet potato

4 scallions, dark, green parts, sliced and divided

½ teaspoon oregano, dried

1 tablespoon garlic oil

2 tablespoons avocado oil, divided

1 organic red bell pepper, diced

Maple-sage breakfast, uncooked (recipe provided)

- Pre-heat your oven to 400 degrees F.
- Take a baking sheet and add sweet potatoes, half of the sliced scallions, oregano, garlic oil, 1 tablespoon avocado oil and mix well
- Mix well and coat the sweet potatoes.
- Bake for 30 minutes.
- Once done, take a large skillet and place it over medium-high heat, add red bell pepper and cook until soft.
- Add sausages and cook for 10 minutes.
- Add sweet potato mixture and mix well until combined thoroughly.
- Divide among four plates and serve, enjoy!

Per Serving: Calories: 330; Total Fat: 24g; Saturated Fat: 5g; Protein: 11g; Carbs: 18g; Fiber: 1g; Sugar: 7g

Creamed up Mashed Potatoes

Servings: 4 / Preparation Time: 10 minutes/ Cooking Time: 20 minutes

Fancy some mashed potatoes but want to add a little bit more zing? This creamy mashed potato is the one to go with!

2 pounds organic white russet potatoes, peeled

8 tablespoons ghee

2/3 cup lactose free milk, warmed

1 teaspoon salt

2 tablespoons fresh chives, chopped

- Add potatoes in a large sized pot and cover it with cold water.
- Place it over high heat and bring to a boil.
- Lower heat to medium-high and cook for 20 minutes until potatoes are tender.
- Use immersion blender (with whisk attachment) and mash the potatoes while adding warm milk.
- Add salt and mix until smooth.
- Serve with topped chives and enjoy!

Per Serving: Calories: 585; Total Fat: 31g; Saturated Fat: 1g; Protein: 9g; Carbs: 71g; Fiber: 0g; Sugar: 6g

Hearty Cinnamon Sweet Potatoes

Servings: 4 / Preparation Time: 5 minutes/ Cooking Time: nil

If you fancy sweet potatoes and want a little bit more flavor, these cinnamon touched sweet potatoes are the ones to go for!

2 cups mashed sweet potatoes, cooked   4 tablespoons ghee

1 teaspoon ground cinnamon

- Take a medium bowl and add sweet potatoes, cinnamon and ghee and mash until well mixed and creamy.
- Serve with your desired toppings and enjoy!

Per Serving: Calories: 194; Total Fat: 15g; Saturated Fat: 5g; Protein: 2g; Carbs: 14g; Fiber: 1g; Sugar: 10g

Cool Cinnamon Rice

Servings: 1 / Preparation Time: 5 minutes/ Cooking Time: 5 minutes

Yet another rice recipe at your service! But this one is dedicated for the Cinnamon lovers out there!

1 cup cooked white rice

1 tablespoon organic grass fed- butter

½ teaspoon ground cinnamon

¼ cup lactose free coconut milk

- Take a microwave safe bowl and add rice, butter, cinnamon, milk and microwave on high for 1 minute until thoroughly heated.
- Serve warm and enjoy!

Per Serving: Calories: 364; Total Fat: 20g; Saturated Fat: 4g; Protein: 2g; Carbs: 42g; Fiber: 1g; Sugar: 3g

Parmesan Polenta Fries

Servings: 2 / Preparation Time: 5 minutes/ Cooking Time: 45 minutes

Many individuals are not familiar with polenta, just give it a try! The cheesy flavors will make you melt.

2 tablespoons olive oil

1 pound polenta

¼ cup parmesan, shredded

- Preheat your oven to 425 degree F.
- Slice a polenta into fries.
- Use olive oil to brush on a baking sheet.
- Bake for 45-50 minutes, turning midway through.
- Serve with parmesan on top.

Per Serving: Calories: 385; Total Fat: 17g; Saturated Fat: 10g; Protein: 17g; Carbs: 41g; Fiber: 2g; Sugar: 10g

Veggie Herbal Quinoa

Servings: 4 / Preparation Time: 30 minutes/ Cooking Time: 10 minutes

It's a really sad fact that many people still hate quinoa! Even though it is possibly one of the healthiest grain out there. Well, this herbed quinoa might just change their perspective!

2 cups quinoa, cooked

2 cups steamed broccoli crowns

2 cups organic cherry tomatoes, halved

1 cup carrots, shredded, steamed

¼ cup fresh basil leaves, chopped

2 tablespoons fresh parsley leaves, chopped

2 tablespoons fresh chives, chopped

2/3 cup extra virgin olive oil

¼ cup white wine vinegar

1 heaping tablespoon Dijon mustard (no garlic)

¼ cup microgreens

- Take a medium bowl and add cooked quinoa, steamed broccoli, tomatoes, carrots, basil, parsley and chives
- Take a blender and add olive oil, vinegar, mustard and blend well.
- Pour dressing over salad and stir well.
- Top salad with microgreens and serve.
- Enjoy!

Per Serving: Calories: 529; Total Fat: 40g; Saturated Fat: 8g; Protein: 12g; Carbs: 37g; Fiber: 2g; Sugar: 8g

_Fancy Stir Fried Quinoa

Servings: 4 / Preparation Time: 5 minutes/ Cooking Time: 20 minutes

Yet another Quinoa dish designed to help change the perspective of the "Non-Believers"! This simple but veggie packed stir fried Quinoa is to diet for!

2 tablespoons coconut oil

1 cup carrot, shredded

1 cup fresh spinach, chopped

2 cups quinoa, cooked

2 cups organic chicken, cooked and chopped

2 teaspoons yellow curry powder

½ cup coconut milk

Salt as needed

- Take a large saucepan and place it over medium-high heat. Add coconut oil and heat up.
- Add carrots, Sauté for 10 minutes.
- Add spinach and cook for 1 minute.
- Stir in cooked quinoa, chicken, curry powder and coconut milk.
- Cook for 5 minutes.
- Season with salt and pepper.
- Serve and enjoy!

Per Serving: Calories: 308; Total Fat: 15g; Saturated Fat: 4g; Protein: 24g; Carbs: 24g; Fiber: 1g; Sugar: 3g

Oven Baked Potato Wedges

Servings: 4 / Preparation Time: 10 minutes/ Cooking Time: 15-20 minutes

Nothing more to say about this dish that you already don't know! The official oven baked potato wedges for your SIBO program!

4 tablespoons olive oil

1 tablespoon thyme, dried

2 large potatoes

Salt and ground black pepper, to taste

- Preheat your oven to 400 degree F.
- Clean and cut potatoes into wedges.
- Toss with salt, thyme, salt and pepper.
- Bake for 15-20 minutes.
- Serve and enjoy!

Per Serving: Calories: 172; Total Fat: 5g; Saturated Fat: 1g; Protein: 2g; Carbs: 31g; Fiber: 1g; Sugar: 6g

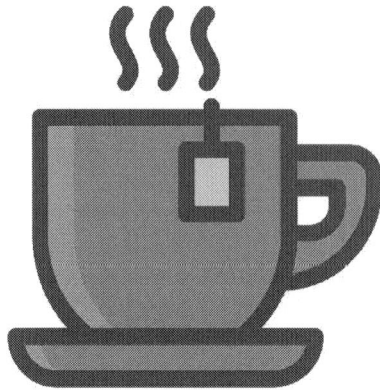

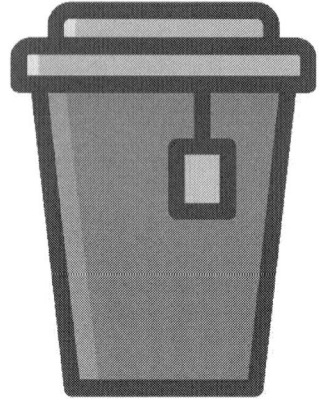

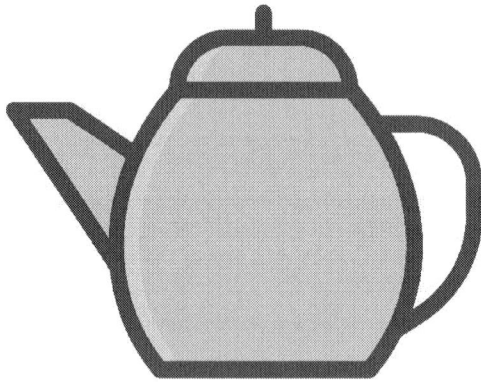

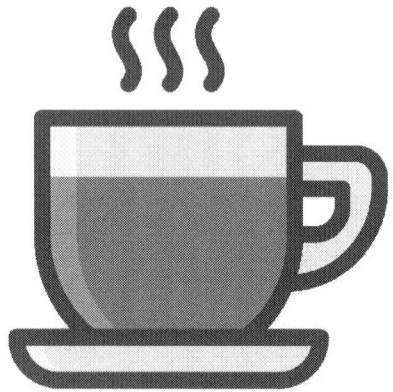

CHAPTER 8: DRINKS AND SNACKS

Contents

SIBO Macaroni & Cheese

Servings: 2 / Preparation Time: 5 minutes/ Cooking Time: 25 minutes

The fan favorite Mac and Cheese now on your SIBO program, prepared to perfection!

1 tablespoon butter

1 tablespoon flour, spelt

4 ounces pasta, gluten free

½ cup milk, lactose-free

Black pepper

1 cup cheese, grated

¼ teaspoon salt

- Take a small saucepan and heat milk over medium heat into it.
- Take another small saucepan then melt butter over medium heat in that pan.
- Add flour when butter starts bubbling.
- Cook when stirring for 1 minute.
- Whisk in the hot milk to the butter-flour mixture.
- Whisk constantly till the mixture is thick and bubbling.
- Remove pan from heat and stir in cheese, salt and pepper.
- Set it aside to cool.
- Cook and drain pasta.
- Boil pasta and add cheese sauce to taste.
- Serve and enjoy!

Per Serving: Calories: 183; Total Fat: 11g; Saturated Fat: 3g; Protein: 6g; Carbs: 14g; Fiber: 1g; Sugar: 2g

Delicious Ginger-Turmeric Tea

Servings: 4 / Preparation Time: 10 minutes/ Cooking Time: 15 minutes

An early morning ginger turmeric tea for all of the moments when you need something to soothe your throat.

4 cups cold water

1 (3 inch) piece fresh turmeric root, peeled and cut into large pieces

1 (3 inch) piece fresh ginger, peeled and cut into large pieces

¼ cup pasteurized clove honey

2 whole cloves

2 star anise

1 cinnamon stick

1 teaspoon peppercorns

½ large lemon, quartered

- Take your blender and add water, turmeric, ginger, blend on high until turmeric and ginger are chopped.
- Transfer to saucepan and place over high heat.
- Add honey, cloves, star anise, cinnamon stick, and peppercorn and bring to a boil. Lower heat to low and simmer for 10 minutes.
- Strain mixture and discard the spices.
- Pour into four mugs and garnish with lemon wedge, enjoy!

Per Serving: Calories: 76; Total Fat: 0g; Saturated Fat: 0g; Protein: 0g; Carbs: 20g; Fiber: 1g; Sugar: 17g

_Ginger Lemonade

Servings: 3 / Preparation Time: 5 minutes/ Cooking Time: nil

Classical lemonade with a gingerly twist! The perfect summer refreshment.

5 cups water

1 cup honey-ginger syrup

¾ cup fresh squeezed lime juice

- Take a large pitcher and stir in water, syrup, and lime juice.
- Adjust the flavor accordingly and chill, serve and enjoy!

Per Serving: Calories: 134; Total Fat: 0g; Saturated Fat: 0g; Protein: 0g; Carbs: 0g; Fiber: 0g; Sugar: 33g

Collection Of Assorted Nuts

Servings: 12 / Preparation Time: 5 minutes/ Cooking Time: 20 minutes

Delicious collection of assorted nuts for any future camping trip!

4 cups raw almonds, macadamia, walnuts, pecans as you desire

3 tablespoons maple syrup

2 tablespoons extra-virgin olive oil

2 tablespoons fresh rosemary, thyme and sage mixture

1 teaspoon smoked paprika

2 teaspoons alt

Fresh ground pepper

- Pre-heat your oven to 350 degrees F.

- Line baking sheet with parchment paper. Add nuts to the sheets alongside syrup, olive oil, herbs, paprika and 2 teaspoons of salt. Season well to taste and mix.

- Bake for 15-20 minutes, making sure to stir twice.

- Remove from oven and stir. Let it cool and serve, enjoy!

Per Serving: Calories: 365; Total Fat: 34g; Saturated Fat: 4g; Protein: 8g; Carbs: 12g; Fiber: 0g; Sugar: 6g

_Cashew And Almond Butter

Servings: 2 / Preparation Time: 5 minutes/ Cooking Time: nil

A hearty almond and cashew flavored butter mix for your SIBO indulgence. .

1 cup almonds, blanched

1/3 cup cashew nuts

2 tablespoons coconut oil

Salt as needed

½ teaspoon cinnamon

- Pre-heat your oven to 350 degree F.
- Bake almonds and cashews for 12 minutes.
- Let them cool.
- Transfer to food processor and add remaining ingredients.
- Add oil and keep blending until smooth.
- Serve and enjoy!

Per Serving: Calories: 168; Total Fat: 13g; Saturated Fat: 4g; Protein: 3g; Carbs: 14g; Fiber: 0g; Sugar: g

Lemon Broccoli Crunchies

Servings: 2 / Preparation Time: 10 minutes/ Cooking Time: 15 minutes

Lemon flavored broccoli florets just the way your Grandma used to make. Prepare to miss your county!

2 heads broccoli, separated into florets

2 teaspoons extra virgin olive oil

1 teaspoon salt

½ teaspoon pepper

½ teaspoon lemon juice

- Pre-heat your oven to a temperature of 400 degree F.
- Take a large sized bowl and add broccoli florets with some extra virgin olive oil, pepper, sea salt.
- Spread the broccoli out in a single even layer on a fine baking sheet.
- Bake in your pre-heated oven for about 15-20 minutes until the florets are soft enough so that they can be pierced with a fork.
- Squeeze lemon juice over them generously before serving.
- Enjoy!

Per Serving: Calories: 130 Total Fat: 10g; Saturated Fat: 3g; Protein: 6g; Carbs: 6g; Fiber: 1g; Sugar: 0g

SIBO Friendly Bread Loaf

Servings: 5 / Preparation Time: 7 minutes/ Cooking Time: 40 minutes

Some people think that you have to abandon bread while you are on your SIBO, this recipe is here to change that perspective!

1 tablespoon sesame seeds

3 tablespoons olive oil

2 teaspoons fresh yeast granules

3 eggs

2 tablespoons sugar

¾ cup tapioca flour

½ cup brown rice flour

1 cup warm water

½ cup potato starch

2 tablespoons chia seeds

1 and ½ cups white rice flour

1 teaspoon salt

1 teaspoon white wine vinegar

- Take a bread maker and add all ingredients into it.
- Set on DOUGH.
- When mixed, oil a loaf tin and place on it.
- Put in the drawer under oven for 30 minutes to keep it warm.
- Preheat your oven to 350 degree F.
- Bake until when top is knocked using a knuckle it sounds hollow or for about 30.
- Allow 5 minutes in the loaf tin and let it cool.
- Serve and enjoy!

Per Serving: Calories: 268; Total Fat: 4g; Saturated Fat: 1g; Protein: 10g; Carbs: 49g; Fiber: 1g; Sugar: 4g

Gnocchi with Lemon & Herb Pesto

Servings: 4 / Preparation Time: 10 minutes/ Cooking Time: 20 minutes

Some people often don't really fancy Gnocchi on its own, the herbed pesto and lemon is here to give you that perfect marriage of flavor!

1 tablespoon garlic infused oil

1 pound pack gluten free gnocchi

Small bunch parsley, finely chopped

4 tablespoons olive oil

1 lemon, zest and juice

2 tablespoons roughly toasted pine nuts, chopped

Snipped small bunch chives

2 tablespoons parmesan, grated

- Take a small bowl, put pine nuts, cheese, lemon zest, herbs and garlic oil and season well.
- Stir in lemon juice and olive oil and keep it aside.
- Take a pan of salted boiling water and cook the gnocchi as per the instructions on the pack and then drain.
- Take a serving bowl and toss into pesto.
- Serve with more parmesan.

Per Serving: Calories: 588; Total Fat: 15g; Saturated Fat: 8g; Protein: 21g; Carbs: 60g; Fiber: 2g; Sugar: 5g

Tender Chicken Chips

Servings: 3 / Preparation Time: 5 minutes/ Cooking Time: 15 minutes

If you are lover of chicken skin, then these chicken skin chips are the ones to die for!

6 organic chicken skins, similar sized

Salt and pepper to taste

Spices such as curry, cumin, chili powder for seasoning

- Pre-heat your oven to 425 degrees F.
- Pat skins dry with paper towels and stretch them on a rimmed baking sheet.
- Sprinkle salt and pepper and other desired spices.
- Bake for 12-15 minutes.
- Once crisp, break in small chunks and serve. Enjoy!

Per Serving: Calories: 259; Total Fat: 23g; Saturated Fat: 2g; Protein: 12g; Carbs: 0g; Fiber: 1g; Sugar: 0g

_Energizing Blueberry-Coconut Milk

Servings: 3 / Preparation Time: 5 minutes/ Cooking Time: nil

Quickly made Blueberry and Coconut Milk drink that has the potential to act as your perfect dessert to end the day!

1 cup organic unsweetened shredded coconut

1 cup blueberries, fresh

6 cups boiling water

1-2 tablespoons clover honey

1-2 teaspoons vanilla extract

- Take a blender and add coconut and blueberries.
- Add boiling water until three-fourths full.
- Add honey and let it sit for 30 minutes until lukewarm.
- Add vanilla and blend on high speed for 1 minute.
- Transfer mixture to nut milk bag and strain the liquid into a bowl.
- Squeeze any liquid out of bag until coconut is mostly dry. Discard solids and transfer milk to a storage container.
- Serve and enjoy!

Per Serving: Calories: 124; Total Fat: 0g; Saturated Fat: 0g; Protein: 1g; Carbs: 8g; Fiber: 0g; Sugar: 6g

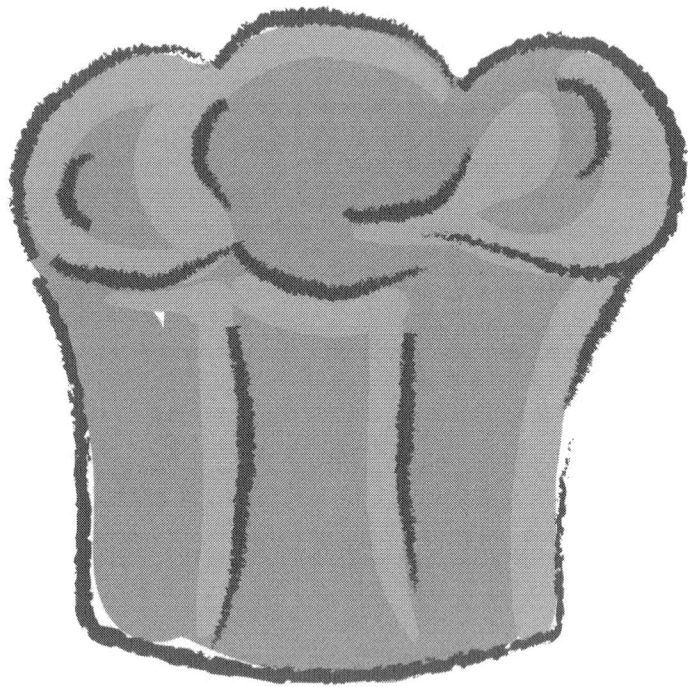

CHAPTER 9: DESSERT

Contents

Chocolate Bark

Servings: 8 / Preparation Time: 2 hours/ Cooking Time: 2 hours

A nice dessert for chocolate lovers who are following the SIBO program, these "Barks" are the perfect dessert for any occasion and any choco lover following the SIBO program.

1 cup cacao butter

¼ stevia, powdered

½ cup hazelnuts

½ cup cacao powder

2 tablespoons pumpkin seeds

½ tablespoon vanilla powder

¾ cup coconut, flaked

- Preheat your oven at 325 degree F.
- Take a baking paper and line a baking sheet and place flaked coconut.
- Take a tray and place it in the oven for 5-10 minutes.
- Once the coconut has toasted then remove it from the oven.
- Set aside.
- Chop the cacao butter in even pieces and place them in the microwave for 1-2 minutes.
- Add vanilla powder and stevia in the melted cacao butter and stir carefully.
- Scrape the thickened chocolate off the baking paper and heat in the microwave for 10-15 seconds.
- Stir properly.
- Take a baking paper and pour the chocolate over it then sprinkle with pumpkin seeds and coconut hazelnuts.
- Place it in the fridge for 5-10 minutes.
- Serve and store the remaining chocolate.

Per Serving: Calories: 234; Total Fat: 14g; Saturated Fat: 7g; Protein: 3g; Carbs: 31g; Fiber: 2g; Sugar: 24g

Rhubarb Roasted Orange

Servings: 4 / Preparation Time: 10 minutes/ Cooking Time: 20 minutes

Initially this might not seem like a dessert, but trust me, the flavors of this dish makes it an awesome amalgam of orangey goodness that makes it one of the best desserts in the business!

1 cup dry vermouth

¼ cup pasteurized clover honey

2 tablespoons fresh squeezed orange juice

Zest of ½ organic orange

8 rhubarb talks, edges trimmed

- Pre-heat your oven to 350 degrees F.
- Take a small bowl and add vermouth, honey, orange juice, orange zest and mix until combined.
- Transfer rhubarb stalks to baking dish and top with vermouth mixture, cover baking dish with foil and bake for 20 minutes until rhubarb softens.
- Enjoy!

Per Serving: Calories: 116; Total Fat: 0g; Saturated Fat: 0g; Protein: 44g; Carbs: 24g; Fiber: 3g; Sugar: 20g

10 Minute Muffin

Servings: 4 / Preparation Time: 5 minutes/ Cooking Time: 10 minutes

Craving muffins in the middle of the night? Just plot up a batch of these in just 10 minutes and be ready to munch on them all night long!

1 tablespoon pasteurized clover honey

2 tablespoons vanilla

1 tablespoon cinnamon

1 ripe banana

½ cup nut butter

¼ teaspoon baking soda

- Preheat your oven to 400 degree F.
- Spray a mini-muffin tin with a cooking spray.
- Add all ingredients into your blender or food processor and blend till mix properly.
- Spoon mixture to the muffin tin.
- Bake for about 10 minutes.
- Let it cool and preserve it in airtight container.
- Serve and enjoy!

Per Serving: Calories: 263; Total Fat: 13g; Saturated Fat: 2g; Protein: 8g; Carbs: 33g; Fiber: 1g; Sugar: 12g

Cool Lemon Mousse

Servings: 4 / Preparation Time: 10 minutes + chill time/ Cooking Time: 10 minutes

Just because you can't have an excess of sweet, doesn't mean that you can't have mousse right? This easy Lemon Mousse is all that you are going to need to have a guilt-free mousse experience.

1 cup coconut cream

8 ounces cream cheese, soft

¼ cup lemon juice

3 pinches salt

- Pre-heat your oven to 350 degree F.
- Grease a ramekin with butter.
- Beat cream, cream cheese, fresh lemon juice, salt in a mixer.
- Pour batter into ramekin.
- Bake for 10 minutes then transfer mouse to serving glass.
- Let it chill for 2 hours and serve.
- Enjoy!

Per Serving: Calories: 241; Total Fat: 20g; Saturated Fat: 3g; Protein: 3g; Carbs: 15g; Fiber: 1g; Sugar: 12g

Matcha Bomb

Servings: 4 / Preparation Time: 10 minutes + chill time/ Cooking Time: nil

A glorious ice bomb for lovers of Green Tea! A healthy and mesmerizing dessert all in one!

¾ cup hemp seeds

½ cup coconut oil

2 tablespoons coconut butter

1 teaspoon Matcha powder

2 tablespoons vanilla bean extract

½ teaspoon mint extract

- Take your blender/food processor and add hemp seeds, coconut oil, Matcha, vanilla extract.
- Blend until you have a nice batter and divide into silicon molds.
- Melt coconut butter and drizzle on top.
- Let the cups chill and enjoy!

Per Serving: Calories: 200; Total Fat: 20g; Saturated Fat: 3g; Protein: 5g; Carbs: 3g; Fiber: 1g; Sugar: 1g

Blueberry Muffins

Servings: 4 / Preparation Time: 10 minutes/ Cooking Time: 20 minutes

Craving for a muffin with a twist? These blueberry packed muffins will completely satisfy your sweet tooth while keeping you guilt free!

1 cup almond flour

Pinch of salt

1/8 teaspoon baking soda

1 whole egg

2 tablespoons coconut oil

½ cup coconut milk

¼ cup fresh blueberries

- Pre-heat your oven to 350 degree F.
- Line a muffin tin with paper muffin cups.
- Add almond flour, salt, baking soda to a bowl and mix, keep it on the side.
- Take another bowl and add egg, coconut oil, coconut milk and mix.
- Add mix to flour mix and gently combine until incorporated.
- Mix in blueberries and fill the cupcakes tins with batter.
- Bake for 20-25 minutes.
- Enjoy!

Per Serving: Calories: 167; Total Fat: 15g; Saturated Fat: 3g; Protein: 5g; Carbs: 3g; Fiber: 1g; Sugar: 1g

Crispy Cheese Balls

Servings: 4 / Preparation Time: 5 minutes/ Cooking Time: 12 minutes

Creative cheesy balls, ready for you to devour and enjoy!

2 eggs, whisked

½ cup almond flour

½ cup cheddar cheese, shredded

12 cup mozzarella cheese, shredded

½ teaspoon baking powder

- Pre-heat your oven to 400 degrees F.
- Add all of the ingredients and mix well.
- Form 8 balls using the mixture and transfer to parchment lined baking sheet.
- Bake for 15-20 minutes.
- Serve and enjoy!

Per Serving: Calories: 213; Total Fat: 16g; Saturated Fat: 6g; Protein: 13g; Carbs: 3g; Fiber: 2g; Sugar: 0g

Hearty Parsley Soufflé

Servings: 4 / Preparation Time: 5 minutes/ Cooking Time: 6 minutes

A hearty soufflé touched with sprinkles of parsley, delicious!

2 whole eggs

1 fresh red chili pepper, chopped

2 tablespoons coconut cream

1 tablespoon fresh parsley, chopped

Salt as needed

- Pre-heat your oven to 390 degree F.
- Butter 2 soufflé dishes.
- Add the ingredients to a blender and mix well.
- Divide batter into soufflé dishes and bake for 6 minutes.
- Serve and enjoy!

Per Serving: Calories: 137; Total Fat: 11g; Saturated Fat: 11g; Protein: 9g; Carbs: 1g; Fiber: 0g; Sugar: 0g

No Bake Fudge

Servings: 3 / Preparation Time2 hours/ Cooking Time: nil

Exuberant coco fudge that can be prepared with absolutely zero baking knowledge!

1 and ¾ cups coconut butter

1 cup pumpkin puree

1 teaspoon ground cinnamon

¼ teaspoon ground nutmeg

1 tablespoon coconut oil

- Take an 8x8 inch square baking pan and line it up with aluminum foil.
- Take a spoon and scoop out coconut butter into a heated pan and allow the butter to melt.
- Keep stirring well and remove the heat once fully melted.
- Add spices and pumpkin and keep straining until you have a grain like texture.
- Add coconut oil and keep stirring to incorporate everything.
- Scoop the mixture into your baking pan and evenly distribute it.
- Place a wax paper on top of the mixture and press gently to straighten the top.
- Remove the paper and discard.
- Allow it to chill for 1-2 hours.
- Once chilled, take it out and slice it up into pieces.
- Enjoy!

Per Serving: Calories: 140; Total Fat: 14g; Saturated Fat: 0g; Protein: 0g; Carbs: 4g; Fiber: 0g; Sugar: 3g

Chocolate Pecan Nut Butter

Servings: 2 cups / Preparation Time: 5 minutes/ Cooking Time: 25 minutes

If you are bored of the traditional peanut butter, this pecan nut butter should satisfy you butter lust!

1 pound raw pecans

1 teaspoon salt

1/3 cup melted dark chocolate

½ teaspoon ground cinnamon

- Pre-heat your oven to 350 degrees F.
- Spread pecans in even layer on rimmed baking sheet and roast for 11 minutes.
- Remove nuts from oven and let them cool for 10 minutes.
- Transfer to food processor and process until buttery.
- Scrape the bottom and sides, add 1 teaspoon salt, chocolate and cinnamon to the processor and blend again.
- Season and use as needed.

Per Serving: Calories: 228; Total Fat: 22g; Saturated Fat: 4g; Protein: 3g; Carbs: 6g; Fiber: 1g; Sugar: 2g

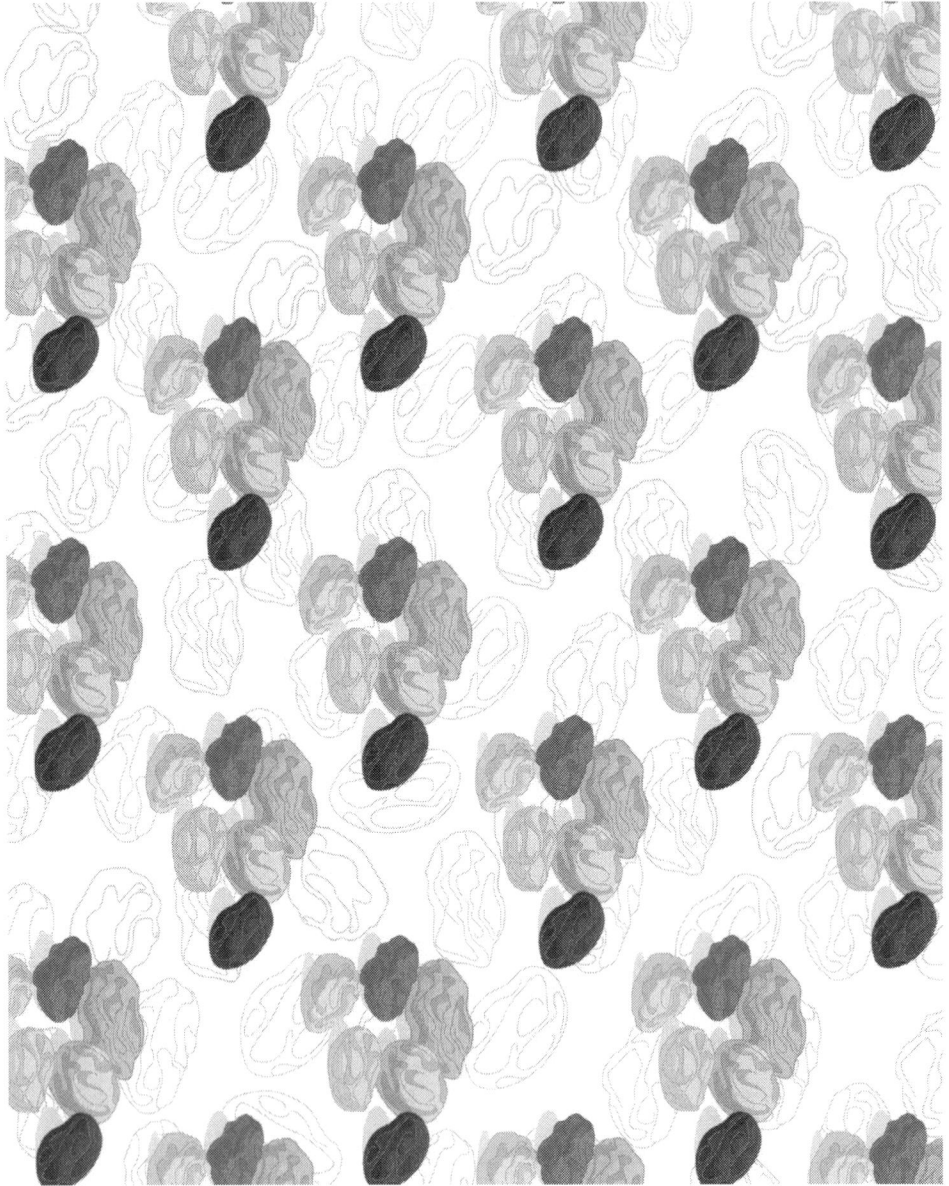

CHAPTER 10: STAPLES, DRESSINGS, CONDIMENTS

Contents

Light Honey And Ginger Syrup

Servings: 1 and ½ cups / Preparation Time: 5 minutes/ Cooking Time: 40 minutes

A fine and sensitive SIBO friendly honey syrup that you can use with any dish to add a captivating touch of flavor to your meals.

1 cup water

1 cup pasteurized clover honey

¼ cup fresh ginger, coarsely chopped, peeled

- Take a small saucepan and place it over high heat, add water, honey and ginger.
- Cook until boiling.
- Lower heat to medium low and simmer for 5 minutes.
- Remove heat and let it cool for 30 minutes.
- Strain the syrup through a mesh strainer and discard ginger.
- Serve when needed and enjoy!

Per Serving: Calories: 84; Total Fat: 0g; Saturated Fat: 1g; Protein: 0g; Carbs: 22g; Fiber: 1g; Sugar: 22g

Hearty Mustard Vinaigrette

Servings: 1 and ½ cups / Preparation Time: 5 minutes/ Cooking Time: 40 minutes

This particular mustard vinaigrette is specifically prepared for the SIBO diet regime that helps you to season your dishes with a nice mustardy flavor.

¼ cup extra virgin olive oil

¼ cup garlic oil

1 and ½ tablespoons red wine vinegar

1 tablespoons fresh squeezed lemon juice

1 rounded tablespoon Dijon mustard

Salt and pepper to taste

- Take a small Mason jar and add olive oil, garlic oil, vinegar, lemon juice, mustard.
- Cover the jar and shake to blend.
- Season with salt and pepper and use when needed.

Per Serving: Calories: 193; Total Fat: 22g; Saturated Fat: 3g; Protein: 0g; Carbs: 0g; Fiber: 1g; Sugar: 0g

Cool Ranch Dressing

Servings: 1 cup / Preparation Time: 10 minutes/ Cooking Time: nil

The original "Ranch" dressing to add a cool and soothing sensation to your dishes!

1 cup 24 Hours Yogurt

¼ cup parmesan cheese, finely grated

2 tablespoons garlic oil

1 tablespoon dried chives, chopped

1 teaspoon dried parsley, chopped

½ teaspoon salt

Fresh ground pepper as needed

- Take a mason jar and add yogurt, parmesan cheese, garlic oil, chives, parsley and salt.
- Season with more salt and pepper if needed.
- Stir well to combine the ingredients.
- Use as needed or keep refrigerated for 1 week,
- Enjoy!

Per Serving: Calories: 28; Total Fat: 3g; Saturated Fat: 1g; Protein: 1g; Carbs: 0g; Fiber: 0g; Sugar: 0g

Brilliant Caesar Dressing

Servings: 2 cups / Preparation Time: 10 minutes/ Cooking Time: nil

If you fancy Caesar Salad, then this is the dressing to go with! The perfect Caesar dressing modified for the SIBO diet. Excellent!

2 large eggs

2 large egg yolks

2 tablespoons fresh squeezed lemon juice

1 teaspoon wild caught anchovy paste

½ teaspoon fresh ground black pepper

¼ teaspoon salt

2 tablespoons organic grass-fed butter, melted

1 cup avocado oil

2 tablespoons garlic oil

¼ cup parmesan cheese, grated

1 teaspoon parsley, chopped

- Take a blender and add eggs, egg yolk, lemon juice, anchovy paste, pepper and salt.
- Blend well until well incorporated.
- While the blender is still running, add avocado oil, garlic oil and keep blending until the mixture is thick.
- Transfer to container and stir in parmesan cheese and parsley.
- Use as needed!

Per Serving: Calories: 175; Total Fat: 19g; Saturated Fat: 2g; Protein: 2g; Carbs: 0g; Fiber: 0g; Sugar: 0g

Coconut Sour Cream

Servings: 4 / Preparation Time: 5 minutes/ Cooking Time: nil

This coconut sour cream is bound to give you a blast from the past!

1 can thick unsweetened coconut milk

1 and ½ tablespoons lemon juice

½ tablespoons apple cider vinegar

1/8 teaspoon salt

- Chill the coconut milk over overnight.

- Flip the can upside and open, skim off any liquid.

- Scrap out the thick cream and add lemon juice, vinegar, and salt.

- Whisk well.

- Use as needed!

Per Serving: Calories: 200; Total Fat: 14g; Saturated Fat: 2g; Protein: 3g; Carbs: 26g; Fiber: 1g; Sugar: 10g

Delicious Home-Made Mayo

Servings: 4 / Preparation Time: 5 minutes/ Cooking Time: nil

Mayonnaise is possibly one of the most fan-favorite condiment/sauce to have around the home! But store-bought Mayo's might break your SIBO diet, the solution therefore is to make your own fancy Mayo and go wild with it!

1 whole egg

½ teaspoon salt

½ teaspoon ground mustard

1 and ¼ cup extra light olive oil

1 tablespoon lemon juice

- Place the egg, ground mustard, salt and ¼ cup of olive oil into a food processor.

- Whirl on low until mixed.

- While the processor is running, drizzle remaining olive oil and keep whirling for 3 minutes.

- Add lemon juice and pulse on low until fully mixed.

- Chill for 30 minutes.

- Use as needed.

Per Serving: Calories: 632; Total Fat: 77g; Saturated Fat: 11g; Protein: 41g; Carbs: 27g; Fiber: 2g; Sugar: 8g

REFERENCES AND RESOURCES

Burgis, J. (2016). Response to strict and liberalized specific carbohydrate diet in pediatric Crohn's disease. *World Journal Of Gastroenterology*, *22*(6), 2111. doi: 10.3748/wjg.v22.i6.2111

Chassaing, B., Koren, O., Goodrich, J., Poole, A., Srinivasan, S., Ley, R., & Gewirtz, A. (2015). Dietary emulsifiers impact the mouse gut microbiota promoting colitis and metabolic syndrome. *Nature*, *519*(7541), 92-96. doi: 10.1038/nature14232

Chedid, V., Dhalla, S., Clarke, J., Roland, B., Dunbar, K., & Koh, J. et al. (2014). Herbal Therapy is Equivalent to Rifaximin for the Treatment of Small Intestinal Bacterial Overgrowth. *Global Advances In Health And Medicine*, *3*(3), 16-24. doi: 10.7453/gahmj.2014.019

Francino, M. (2016). Antibiotics and the Human Gut Microbiome: Dysbioses and Accumulation of Resistances. *Frontiers In Microbiology*, *6*. Doi: 10.3389/fmicb.2015.01543

Gearry, R., Skidmore, P., O'Brien, L., Wilkinson, T., & Nanayakkara, W. (2016). Efficacy of the low FODMAP diet for treating irritable bowel syndrome: the evidence to date. *Clinical And Experimental Gastroenterology*, 131. doi: 10.2147/ceg.s86798

Ghoshal, U., Shukla, R., & Ghoshal, U. (2017). Small Intestinal Bacterial Overgrowth and Irritable Bowel Syndrome: A Bridge between Functional Organic Dichotomy. *Gut And Liver*, *11*(2), 196-208. doi: 10.5009/gnl16126

Haskey, N., & Gibson, D. (2017). An Examination of Diet for the Maintenance of Remission in Inflammatory Bowel Disease. *Nutrients*, *9*(3), 259. doi: 10.3390/nu9030259

Kim, S. (2010). Small Intestinal Bacterial Overgrowth. *Intestinal Research*, *8*(2), 106. doi: 10.5217/ir.2010.8.2.106

Kruis, W., Forstmaier, G., Scheurlen, C., & Stellaard, F. (1991). Effect of diets low and high in refined sugars on gut transit, bile acid metabolism, and bacterial fermentation. *Gut*, *32*(4), 367-371. doi: 10.1136/gut.32.4.367

Magnusson, K. (2015). Fat, sugar cause bacterial changes that may relate to loss of cognitive function. Retrieved from http://today.oregonstate.edu/archives/2015/jun/fat-sugar-cause-bacterial-changes-may-relate-loss-cognitive-function

Martins, V., Toledo Florêncio, T., Grillo, L., Do Carmo P. Franco, M., Martins, P., & Clemente, A. et al. (2011). Long-Lasting Effects of Undernutrition. *International Journal Of Environmental Research And Public Health*, *8*(6), 1817-1846. doi: 10.3390/ijerph8061817

Quigley, E., & Quera, R. (2006). Small Intestinal Bacterial Overgrowth: Roles of Antibiotics, Prebiotics, and Probiotics. *Gastroenterology*, *130*(2), S78-S90. doi: 10.1053/j.gastro.2005.11.046

Sheikh, K. (2017). How Gut Bacteria Tell Their Hosts What to Eat. *Scientific American Mind*, *28*(4), 4-6. doi: 10.1038/scientificamericanmind0717-4

SIBO Survivor- Heal Your Gut and Get Back to Living Normally Again!. Retrieved from https://sibosurvivor.com/

Sigall-Boneh, R., Levine, A., Lomer, M., Wierdsma, N., Allan, P., & Fiorino, G. et al. (2017). Research Gaps in Diet and Nutrition in Inflammatory Bowel Disease. A Topical Review by D-ECCO Working Group [Dietitians of ECCO]. *Journal Of Crohn's And Colitis*, *11*(12), 1407-1419. doi: 10.1093/ecco-jcc/jjx109

Staudacher, H. (2017). Nutritional, microbiological and psychosocial implications of the low FODMAP diet. *Journal Of Gastroenterology And Hepatology*, *32*, 16-19. Doi: 10.1111/jgh.13688

Zhong, C., Qu, C., Wang, B., Liang, S., & Zeng, B. (2017). Probiotics for Preventing and Treating Small Intestinal Bacterial Overgrowth. *Journal Of Clinical Gastroenterology*, *51*(4), 300-311. doi: 10.1097/mcg.0000000000000814

THE "DIRTY DOZEN" AND "CLEAN 15"

Every year, the Environmental Working Group releases a list of the produce with the most pesticide residue (Dirty Dozen) and a list of the ones with the least **chance of having residue (Clean 15). It's based on analysis from the U.S.** Department of Agriculture Pesticide Data Program report.

The Environmental Working Group found that 70% of the 48 types of produce tested had residues of at least one type of pesticide. In total there were 178 different pesticides and pesticide breakdown products. This residue can stay on veggies and fruit even after they are washed and peeled. All pesticides are toxic to humans and consuming them can cause damage to the nervous system, reproductive system, cancer, a weakened immune system, and more. Women who are pregnant can expose their unborn children to toxins through their diet, and continued exposure to pesticides can affect their development.

This info can help you choose the best fruits and veggies, as well as which ones you should always try to buy organic.

The Dirty Dozen

- Strawberries
- Spinach
- Nectarines
- Apples
- Peaches
- Celery
- Grapes
- Pears
- Cherries
- Tomatoes
- Sweet bell peppers
- Potatoes

The Clean 15

- Sweet corn
- Avocados
- Pineapples
- Cabbage
- Onions
- Frozen sweet peas
- Papayas
- Asparagus
- Mangoes
- Eggplant
- Honeydew
- Kiwi
- Cantaloupe
- Cauliflower
- Grapefruit

MEASUREMENT CONVERSION TABLES

VOLUME EQUIVALENTS (DRY)

US Standard	Metric (Approx.)
¼ teaspoon	1 ml
½ teaspoon	2 ml
1 teaspoon	5 ml
1 tablespoon	15 ml
¼ cup	59 ml
½ cup	118 ml
1 cup	235 ml

WEIGHT EQUIVALENTS

US Standard	Metric (Approx.)
½ ounce	15 g
1 ounce	30 g
2 ounces	60 g
4 ounces	115 g
8 ounces	225 g
12 ounces	340 g
16 oz or 1 lb	455 g

VOLUME EQUIVALENTS (LIQUID)

US Standard	US Standard (ounces)	Metric (Approx.)
2 tablespoons	1 fl oz	30 ml
¼ cup	2 fl oz	60 ml
½ cup	4 fl oz	120 ml
1 cup	8 fl oz	240 ml
1 ½ cups	12 fl oz	355 ml
2 cups or 1 pint	16 fl oz	475 ml
4 cups or 1 quart	32 fl oz	1 L
1 gallon	128 fl oz	4 L

OVEN TEMPERATURES

Fahrenheit (F)	Celsius (C) (Approx)
250°F	120°C
300°F	150°C
325°F	165°C
350°F	180°C
375°F	190°C
400°F	200°C
425°F	220°C
450°F	230°C

30 DAY SIBO DIET PLAN

Qty	Breakfast	Lunch	Dinner
1	Hearty Maple Sage Breakfast	Crisp Spiced Chicken	Lemony Shrimp Rice
2	Kale And Avocado Skillet	Salmon And Spinach Bake	Healthy Broccoli And Lemon Butter
3	Stir-Fry Breakfast	Veggie Herbal Quinoa	Hearty Pork Chops With Chimichurri
4	Jalapeno Scrambled Eggs	Sesame Beef	Chili Chicken
5	Lovely Devilled Eggs	Awesome Mahi-Mahi And Avocado Lime	Hearty Cinnamon Sweet Potatoes
6	Traditional Scrambled Eggs	Pesto Turkey Meatballs	Herb-Crusted Fish
7	Pumpkin Pancakes	Mushroom Pork Chops	Delicious Easy Steak
8	Scrambled Up Pesto Eggs	Sweet Roasted Maple Parsnips	Original Carrot Puree
9	Cheesy Omelet	Almond Coated Chicken	Peri Peri Chicken
10	Grain Free Breakfast Oatmeal	Slowly Cooked Lamb Curry	All-Time Favorite Zucchini Chips
11	Stir-Fry Breakfast	Salmon Lemon Fish Cakes	Homely Lamb Chops
12	Hearty Maple Sage Breakfast	Cool Hearty Baked Eggplant	Simple Baked White Fish
13	Lovely Devilled Eggs	Baked Salmon with Potatoes	Avocado Beef Patties
14	Pumpkin Pancakes	Beef Sauté And Zucchini With Coriander	Black Berry Chicken Wings
15	Cheesy Omelet	Fancy Stir Fried Quinoa	Tender Sweet Potato Hash
16	Jalapeno Scrambled Eggs	Fancy Asian Ground Pork Ala Lettuce Cups	Hearty Pork Chops With Chimichurri
17	Traditional Scrambled Eggs	Baked Parmesan Chicken	Pork Rinds In Stick
18	Scrambled Up Pesto Eggs	Parmesan Polenta Fries	Lovely Bacon Wrapped Chicken Livers
19	Grain Free Breakfast Oatmeal	Creamed up Mashed Potatoes	Avocado Beef Patties

20	Kale And Avocado Skillet	Salmon with Green Bean Salad	Baked Salmon with Potatoes
21	Lovely Devilled Eggs	Brussels Platter	Oven Baked Potato Wedges
22	Grain Free Breakfast Oatmeal	Lemon Basil Chicken Dish	Tender Poached Chicken Breast
23	Pumpkin Pancakes	Eat Butter with Avocado and Smoked Salmon	All Time Favorite Spinach Sautee
24	Traditional Scrambled Eggs	Simple Delight Bruschetta	Simple Baked White Fish
25	Scrambled Up Pesto Eggs	French Oven Beef Stew	Warm Swiss Chard
26	Cheesy Omelet	Zucchini BBQ	Sesame Beef
27	Hearty Maple Sage Breakfast	Dill And Potato Delight	Leeks Platter
28	Stir-Fry Breakfast	Super Easy Oven Baked Chicken	Chicken And Zucchini Zoodles
29	Kale And Avocado Skillet	Great Tomato And Garlic Shrimp	Delicious Easy Steak
30	Jalapeno Scrambled Eggs	Parmesan Herb Rice	Cool Cinnamon Rice

INDEX

22429598R00093

Printed in Great Britain
by Amazon